MS YOU DON'T OWN ME

ONE WOMAN'S APPROACH TO OVERCOMING MULTIPLE SCLEROSIS NATURALLY

MARIA ANN LAVER

Second edition 2025

***

ISBN 978-1-78792-092-7

Front cover: Photo Credit: Scott Dunleavy

Internal Author Photo Credit: Andreea Tufescu

Book design, layout and production management by Into Print
www.intoprint.net
+44 (0)1604 832149

DEDICATION

This book is dedicated to my two beautiful children who
I love very much.

***

CONTENTS

ACKNOWLEDGEMENTS

This book is about how I have learnt to live with MS. I did that with the help and encouragement of many people, some of whom I would like to take the space here to thank:

My mother, Victoria who is my rock, and has always believed in me. To her I shall be eternally grateful.

Lucille Bramble, a close friend of 41 years, who sadly passed away while I was writing this book. An incredible woman with an insatiable zest for life. May she fly high like a butterfly.

Kay Dawn Lock, who passed away in 2009, aged 46, with ovarian cancer. She was a dear friend, my work partner in crime at the Automobile Association and the Godmother to my children.

Phyllis Thornhill, a friend for 32 years and Godmother to my children. In all those years we have never had a cross word. Christine Mattan, a friend and former neighbour. She assisted with my lumber puncture in 2012 and has also been my beauty therapist. Christine was there for me at a very difficult time in my life.

Carole Day, who has been a good friend, never judges me and is there for me in times of need.

My path also crossed two incredible people, Frank Blaney and his lovely wife, Collette Gee. They have guided and helped me to make this book a reality. I really could not have done this without you both.

*****

FOREWORD

As a personal friend and colleague of Maria I have often been immensely inspired by her passion, courage, and genuine kindness. She is a rare gem of a person. It was an honour to assist her in the editing and publishing of this amazing testimony of her approach in confronting this disease that afflicts so many. Far too many. We share her hope and dream that this book will have a massive positive impact on sufferers of MS and other auto-immune disorders. It will have a massive positive impact on not only the victims of MS, but also their caregivers, families, and loved ones. This is a family struggle. As a professional Self-Care and Qigong expert I have trained many organizations and medical support groups over the years. The symptoms Maria describes here would fit many of the countless other auto-immune disorders that are all too prevalent in modern society. Though as she states clearly, everyone's journey of healing is personal and unique. There is something here for everyone to learn. I have seen the significant shift in Maria's well-being and mobility since I have known her. I have seen this amazing change with my own eyes. Though her presence and spirit has always been beautiful and strong, her body was really struggling when we first met. She was walking very slowly, at times with 'sticks'. When I saw her six months or so later she was walking normally. We even took a long train trip into London and wandered around there for a quite a while. I was amazed at the difference within a relatively short period of time in her strength and mobility. All from simple lifestyle changes making a positive impact cumulatively, day by day. Amazing. Seeing what she has accomplished first-hand with my own eyes made me a believer. These are not fanciful, faddish, new 'theories' Maria is sharing. She is simply going back to the older, healthier ways of how our ancestors ate, worked and lived. She went back to the basics. And, it is healing her. Maria Ann Laver invites you to join her in this journey towards deeper wellness and well-being. If it bothers you to not have a specific note referencing a fact or opinion that Maria shares in the book and you need to see a lot of fine print footnotes and endnotes to be impressed by an author's expertise, then this is not the right book for you. You picked up the wrong reading material. Maria read through numerous books like those to learn the information she shares. There are numerous books and journals out there like that. This is purposefully not one of them. Few laypersons have the patience or desire to wade through research journals, thick medical textbooks, endless footnotes, and the like. This book is intended for laypersons who want to learn some simple tools to improve their health and well-being. To learn it in a quick and easy format. This is that book. This book is primarily the testimony of one woman desperately and diligently seeking a solution to her personal health crisis. She put in countless hours deeply researching the information she shares. Even more importantly, she has incorporated every positive exercise, dietary change, and recipe that she shares into her everyday life.

Frank Blaney

***

Transformation

All of our most difficult and profound journeys begin with only one step, followed slowly by one other. I invite you to begin your unique journey to a healthier and happier life. It is really quite simple. We step onto the new ground and by necessity – leave old ground behind. We will leave many things behind on this journey – dead habits that no longer served us. We will bravely try new things, retain what we like and by this grow fresh new wings. Choose this day to fly.
Come Fly.

***

1: A POSITIVE SOLUTION

Why I Wrote This Book

Each morning that I wake is a good morning and one where I am ready to start the day with the biggest challenge of my entire life. I have faced many, as you will learn, but none as monstrous as battling this dreadful disease of Multiple Sclerosis, or 'MS'.

This is a book for *everyone*, especially those who have been diagnosed with Multiple Sclerosis, or any number of neurological disorders; diseases of the brain, spine and nerves that connect within our bodies. It may even be helpful for those who suffer from other auto-immune disorders, of which MS is just one.

This book is also for MS sufferers' family members, friends and caregivers. You need to know first-hand the demons we wrestle with each day, each morning. The families of MS sufferers experience many ups and downs, changes and pragmatic challenges. This is for you all, too. So that you can better understand and cope with our changes, and better adjust to the roller coaster you are riding along with us.

I wrote this book to inspire people to take as many positive steps as possible to control their own illness. I was compelled to share how I have reversed the effects of my illness through my food choices and exercise. I am not preaching, I am sharing what worked for me.

I defeat MS by my will and how I seek to laugh in the face of this adversity – *my* adversity. I want my little victories and blessings to spill over to the many others that struggle with this dreadful disease. We need all the tools and resources we can get to carry on this battle.

I Conspire to Inspire

YOU can do this! We are a community and we can do this together. As a community, we can better manage Multiple Sclerosis (MS).

We can bring back the *joy* in our lives, the *energy*, like we have had previously, the fun times, the laughter. If you cannot laugh at yourself, I feel a bit sorry for you. I know from experience; laughter is far easier than crying. While MS is no joke, the situations you find yourself in sometimes are truly hilarious.

Writing this has been very difficult for me, for various reasons. I do not however, have a problem with talking. Anyone that knows me would gladly confirm this. My brother once said, "I bet your jaws jump for joy when you go to sleep at night, Sis."

"Cheeky Sod, I don't have to like you," I said, "shame we can't choose our family. Ha!" Brotherly love, but family is a source of strength we can lean on through a health crisis.

I have so much I feel I must share. But, it can be summarized by this one fact I feel in my bones; '*YOU are not going to drag me down, MS!*'

It seems like the universe knew all along that this would be my troubled journey. This book relays the *beginning* of my life with MS, *not* the end. I can feel it in my bones. I *am* victorious. I WILL survive this and I will THRIVE in spite of this.

"This is not the end. It is not even the beginning of the end. But it is, perhaps the end of the beginning," – Winston Churchill.

I try to lead by example, having always been a leader and seldom a follower. I will not be controlled, even if I had to let go of my attachments. You are your own person in this life. Accept that truth, that responsibility.

It is only up to you to do what needs to be done. Our beloved Doctors, pharmacists, holistic healers, nurses, and family do not have the ability or responsibility to 'save' us. We must fix ourselves.

You are responsible for yourself and your own actions. Only YOU can change *you!* Remember, when you point your finger at anyone else, take a look at the other three fingers that are pointing back at you.

How I Came to This Point – Love is Powerful

I love the people that I have met through having MS and thoroughly enjoy networking and meeting new people. I do not feel as alone as I did when I first received my diagnosis.

In the beginning I felt totally lost. Fortunately, I no longer feel so isolated. This may sound strange, but we *share* each other's illnesses. We fully understand what each of us are going through and know that we are only a phone call away. I like to make people smile just as others have made me smile.

So many good friends and family have crossed my path. The greatest support is to bring people together from all over the world. We are more connected than ever. But, we are probably the loneliest now, more than ever for the aeons of time humans have been here. This world of technology we live in today, is it truly connecting us?

Many people work from home in their own living room on their computer 24/7. Connecting through Facebook, Twitter, Instagram, etc. Is that a real connection? Are we truly supporting one another in this journey? In this battle?

I see the shape of an open book. It opens outwards to have a good story to tell. There is a wealth of opportunity to help others with these everyday battles I have been through. We all have a book in us to write. We all have a story to tell. What is your story?

This book I have written is part of my life's successes and challenges raising my children and my life journey as a working mother. It has bit of humour, because that is how I deal with life. I cannot help but joke, as you will see. I do not use too much technical jargon. The idea is to get straight to the point and share some helpful tools with you.

MS is a global illness. Hopefully one day this book will be translated into other languages to help those who suffer. Hopefully it will touch people in countries where some people feel alienated and are not reached. My aim is to help improve the lives of other suffers and inspire people to take action – to change their lives for the better.

I have always written in diaries and journals for the last 30 years. Being 'old school', I use the pen and paper. The pen is mightier than the sword! This is a quote I had heard somewhere through my reading when I was younger. I never quite knew what this meant as a child but, I do now. I realize it now.

Thankfully, my editor and the publisher were able to translate my story into an electronic format so that it can be spread the world over to encourage others. I also pecked away as best as I could on the computer keyboard to get the word out.

So here we have what I can humbly offer. I trust it will be a blessing to you. It will be an encouragement to you to make the strongest and best choices possible for your life, health, and future.

The written word exists forever. Whispers and chatter just blow away in the wind and are lost forever. Stories that need to be told need to be set solid with ink upon paper. This is my offering to help encourage you on your journey. Let's do this!

I am happy enough to be dedicated to my health, in a disciplined and controlled way, of working with my own body's inner cells. At the end of the day, they are *mine*. I have had them all my life. They are my responsibility to repair.

I am sharing the choices and tools that helped to stabilized my own body – *without* prescribed medication. Your body does change every seven years, so perhaps your food should change to go with your new chemistry.

There is a saying, "Once a lady, twice a baby" or, "Once a man, twice a child." Everything changes. Nothing remains the same. We have to adapt if we are to survive and thrive.

Your body is a reflection of your lifestyle. Having Multiple Sclerosis, and Osteoporosis together – they seemed to have joined hand in hand and together they took over my body.

I have been coping with my emotional feelings and internal struggles, as well as with my physiological joint pain and decreased mobility. The one–two punch. This is a story of my fight for physical and mental freedom over this dreaded disease, MS.

Personal things are shared in this book. Being a private person, it has been a challenge being so forward about my personal life. Yet, it is important for me to share my life's illness with you now. We can all learn from each other.

I have overcome my pain, to the point of stabilizing lesions in my brain. They are still there, but are not active, or live. What I share here in these pages has really worked for me. I am no one special, but if it worked for me, it can work for you.

The sooner you start to get onboard with better nutrition and an active lifestyle, the sooner you will enjoy the health benefits. You are capable of more than you know. *You can get stronger.*

Cultivating Belief in Yourself

My message to you if you have just been diagnosed with MS – do not be scared! Get onboard, there is hope if you believe in yourself. Self-Belief is very profound. It will empower you and give you more self-esteem and confidence. You are going to need all of that, every day in this battle against MS.

Through action, dedication, determination and willpower you can become free. Having a positive mental attitude will lead to success. I do believe that the hard work will not kill you, it will just make you stronger. This battle is, as you know, *hard* work. But we can encourage each other as we move forward.

My hope is that this book will be translated into many languages and extended around the world one day, because I have experienced first-hand that it works. If worked for me, it can work for others.

You can become better slowly just by integrating a few life changes. To be honest, I do not have a choice of having or not having MS. It is here – my constant unwelcome companion.

Little did I know before being diagnosed with MS I would write this testimony. I did not know or believe I could stabilize my illness. Yet, I have. With simple logical changes in lifestyle. That is something you can control.

Multiple Sclerosis is an illness that has no cure as of yet, but it can be stabilized with a healthy diet and exercise. I have personally experienced the power of this approach. This is why I am here to share my story. Let us take this journey together – hand in hand.

2: WORKING MOTHER'S BLUES

Who I Am

May I digress somewhat and share a bit about my life? I am pulling back the veil of my illness for all to see, so it may be helpful to learn a little more about me.

I was born in the Mid-1960'S to two young parents in their late teenage years, Victoria Hodges, and David Laver and I was christened under the name, Maria Ann Laver. Born in late November, 1964, I was born three weeks late and I have been late ever since, as my brothers would say. They would joke when meeting up for dinner, "Are we on Maria's time today, or on our time?"
They torment the life out of their only sister, cheeky beggars that they are. I thought in this world we are supposed to look up to our elders, aren't we?

I attended the local, secondary modern school in Kent, England. I Left Gordon Secondary School in 1981 and then attended college. I loved (and still love) cooking. I took my two years in the big city of London and joined the Cook's Guild. I was looking for a career as a chef in catering. I worked as a cook and as a 'silver service' waitress in restaurants in London while I attended college.

Studying hard at college and saving my money for my cooking uniforms and chef knives – that was my busy life as a young woman. One week just rolled into another. Weekends would just disappear. I worked hard in many restaurants all over London.

Weekdays I was back at college. From Monday morning to Friday afternoon, time flew very quickly as I studied for my exams. I also worked hard on my social skills to make it successfully in the competitive catering industry.

I grew up with just one parent, my mother. It was very hard to make ends meet.

Learning home-cooking fascinated me. It all grew from there, and the genetic roots were deep. My mother was a cook at West Hill, & Joyce Green Hospitals in Dartford, and also cooked professionally in the working-class town of Gravesend also. My grandparent was also a cook. That passion seems to run through our family genes.

We also have an actor in our family. A dancer also, on my grandmother's family side. We had a little bit of talent, may I say from our family tree going back to the 1700's. From cooking, to acting, singing, and dancing. Quite a talented family.

Working Class Women Wear Many Hats

I mentioned in the introduction that I was a working mother. I come from a working class of people outside of the big city of London. Seeing my mother raise us all by herself, I knew our life start was not easy.

I knew even as a young woman, I would have to work very hard to make ends meet. Some of the crazy jobs I ended up having! But each played their part in making me who I am.

Chef & Professional Cake Baker

To gain experience and earn some pin money I went on to learn Caribbean cooking. I never knew at the time, but this was to be the culture of my future precious children – Afro-Caribbean. My beautiful children help give me strength to press on.

To further my catering career, I moved on to train specifically in cake baking. I loved it and there was descent money in baking delicacies. I attended night school for cake decorating, learning royal sugar icing to cake icing. I was a royal, certified Cake Artist!

I had moved onto making *sugar flowers*, all edible and enjoyable. It was incredible the things you could make from sugar icing. They looked so real after the endless hours that went into the art, design, and modelling of the cakes.

Hair Artist

I also had an interest in doing hair. Not necessarily in cutting hair, although I did learn to cut hair. I became a *hair artist* – in all styles, Afro-Caribbean hair braiding, plaiting and extensions.

It became a craze, in the 80's. My clientele grew out of control. First in Kent, then all around England as word of my hair artist skills spread, even to the newspapers. I got calls and clients all the way from London to Birmingham and even Scotland.

Then finally my clients travelled to catch me at my home. There was a famous film from 1979, the movie '10'. That famous film set the trajectory for 'hip style' braided hair for the whole 80's decade. Everyone wanted that Bo Derek look so that film gave me another unexpected career. Not bad for a working class girl!

Fashion Model

Then One day I auditioned for a fashion show. It went up from catwalk fashion shows onto glamour modelling. From modelling to promotion work – it is funny the odd paths life takes you on.

I even got a gig as a 'Bunny Girl' at the famous Stringfellows Night Club in London's Covent Garden, seeing guests to their tables. I could not believe I had lucked out so much for a humble girl from Kent.

I was headhunted to work for the double glazing company, *Astral Windows* – promotion work to sell plastic PVC windows back in the early 1980's. Not as glamorous, but it paid well.

Road Sales

I walked across a road one day to meet a friend at a work stand in the Whitgift Shopping Centre in Croydon. My friend Ruth was working for the Royal Automobile Club (RAC) motoring organization at the Shopping Centre. She asked me to cover the booth while she went to the loo.

While she was gone I made a couple of sales. My life only got better from there. After signing-up two new members for roadside assistance while I was just watching her stand, I was asked to work for the company. Ruth became my manager a few years later and we became very close friends.

It was a fantastic employment package with a company car and basic salary, commission, fuel card, and a company pension. It was endless luncheon vouchers and wonderful paid holidays around the world on target incentives.

It was ridiculous wages; a license to print money. This was long before the internet and mobile phones, when there were red telephone boxes on the street corner and you had to stand and wait in line to use the phone.

We later got the early mobile phone which was big as a brick. I certainly would not like to have dropped one on my feet. I would have wound up doing a 'Lindy Hop'!

Mortgage Free at 21 Years Old

I bought my first property age twenty in 1984, a small Studio Flat. In just over a year, I had paid off my mortgage. I was mortgage free at twenty-one. Those early learned skills in managing money came in quite handy when all the medical bills started rolling in from the testing and medical visits with the MS.

Finally, after nine years I rented out my property in 1995. I then bought a house. During this time, I was headhunted again for another motoring organization called the Automobile Association (AA). I never had job interview in my entire life!

So I started working full time for the Automobile Association. Within six months I had achieved the year's sales target. I was interviewed by the press as the number one top sales woman – while I was pregnant!

Life Will Slow You Down – One Way or Another

I worked extremely long hours (to an unhealthy degree) for many years for these two different motoring organizations until I was forced to retire due to my illness. Remember, at the end of the day you are just a number. It is tough being a working mother; always having to go the extra mile to make ends meet and keep food on the table.

I had nothing, nothing left for myself. I gave everyone else (including my employers) 100% of my life. When I came home, it was to work for my children and in the evening work for my partner. *Everybody* and *everything* came before me. I was at the bottom. That was not a bad thing, as long as I still had a moment for myself, but I had just stopped having that moment for far too long.

Life at that time truly seemed like a blur, like brain fog; sometimes a cloudy haze. It was like a depersonalization disorder; feeling unreal, detached, and often unable to even *feel* emotion.

After my diagnosis of MS, being unable to work and perhaps further my career – it all came to a full stop. I felt emotional numbness – disconnected from myself.

By dislocating the 'self' from the physical body and its actions, your body is actually protecting your core from further harm. Nature is wonderful in how it protects us.

Depersonalization is most commonly the result of very high anxiety levels. I was truly left feeling like a robot, yet even today, doctors do not really recognize this. It is like a life on autopilot; the absence of emotions, either good or bad. My body and limbs felt as if they were separated. They were no longer my own.

MS symptoms can all be so different. Some people say it is like the wheels are going around on the car, but the cars not moving. For example, the brain is still fully alert to move your limbs, but due to the severed nerve ends caused by the MS, it causes one's limbs to become heavy and limp. They seize up especially after a long haul, like a jet flight over ten hours. This is why I arrange for wheel chair assistance when booking my flights.

Many of you may experience some form of extreme fatigue or high stress simply from not being able to move about. All you want to achieve is just to be able to walk normally again. It causes such deep upset and frustration. To have something you have done all your life be taken away all of a sudden.

We Work and Heal Within Families

It can be hard to deal with for our family members. My thoughts were – *I have got to get a grip of myself, and find a way of feeling well, to the best of my ability.* Especially when I learned more about MS, I understood that I could lose all of my independence one day.

When I was diagnosed with MS, I made a decision. I just did not want to take medication for the rest of my life. I wanted to prove I could stabilize my health through a healthy diet that was natural and avoided processed food. So instead of medication, I committed to eating healthily, dairy free and to engage in regular exercise.

Think about this. If food can make you sick, then reversing your habits can make you well. The whole family can do this together. You can write down in the first month on a chart to make it fun, everything everyone eats. Make it like a game to see who gives in and have an award at the end!

Life is complicated and difficult enough, so make it fun to eat well and achieve great health. As a family trying this, it can be fun together. MS does affect every family member and they are a big part of your healing journey.

My hope is that future generations will not have to go through this chronic, disabling disease of MS. My hope is that we are getting closer to a cure. That is why I have chosen to donate a portion of my profits towards my charities that address MS. Every little bit helps so they can further the necessary research.

What the Hell is Multiple Sclerosis?

The roots of MS still remain a mystery up to this day. Yet, the medical community does see some surprising trends. MS is most common in regions far from the equator. Such as Scandinavia, and other parts of Northern Europe. These places get less sunlight. Most likely, the sunlight (or lack of it) is part of the mystery. They get more demyelinating of inflammation, as well as many other, neurological diseases.

Myelin is a lipid-rich (fatty) substance formed in the central nervous system (CNS) by glial cells called oligodendrocytes, and in the peripheral nervous system (PNS). Only the CNS is affected by MS, when an abnormal immune system response attacks the Myelin sheaths of the nerves.

The Western world has more Parkinson's, Alzheimer's and strokes. When the brain, spinal cord, and nerves get afflicted, that is a dreadful thing. These make up your nervous system. So when something goes wrong there, you can have trouble – with your mobility, speaking, swallowing, seeing and even breathing.

I wanted to share with you a few statistics. I have researched in the books, journals, and in the countries I have travelled. What I have learned along the way has shocked me. Something is going on with neurological diseases and diet.

There are more than 600 diseases afflicting the nervous system. Parkinson's and Alzheimer's disease are well-known, as are strokes, brain tumours, epilepsy, etc. These are just a common few and these can be very frightening when they occur. I wonder sometimes what God has got in store for me. I fight hard to make the best of all this. It is still scary sometimes.

Prevention is better than cure. Our generation and our children's generation are living longer due to science and research. Would you not rather live into a grand old age, or any age while having a healthy life?

Some people would say ignorance is bliss – they would rather not know if they are ill. Whereas my motto is, 'A stitch in time saves nine.' We do have an opportunity to resist this disease. There is no shadow of a doubt that this disabling disease of Multiple Sclerosis can be stabilized.

3: THE BLIND LEADING THE BLIND

Not So Merry Christmas

There was a tension across my forehead with deep pain still in my right eye socket. I felt sick in my stomach. I put this down to being just a headache, but with terrifically intense pain.

My right eye was still hurting. I rubbed my left eye. Then, *the room went completely black.* That is when I went temporarily blind. It was the first time I noticed my sight had gone out in my right eye.

This occurred during Christmas day of 1997, the Christmas holiday when my eyesight disappeared. 'Spastic Hemiplegia,' was the official diagnosis eventually. I had Optic neuritis, but did not know it yet. I was cooking Christmas dinner for 20 family guests and nursing a mean headache with intense pain in my right eye socket. My son was only 20 months old.

We lived at 50 Lennox Road, in Gravesend, England. I was looking forward to Christmas day, but I could have done without this nasty present though. Being a chef by trade, on Christmas Eve I was preparing the food, I loved cooking.

I made Christmas cakes to order. I sold plenty and the orders got bigger year by year. Cooking always – curry goat, and ackee salt fish, turkey, beef, and even lamb. Lots of festive traditional English and Caribbean holiday foods.

As I was busy in the kitchen cooking, the pain in my right eye socket was becoming excruciating for me. It was settling in, letting me know it was here to stay for the holiday. Yet, I had to carry on with the duties of the day. On that Christmas morning I was feeling so blessed to have this wonderful home filled with family. I would always give thanks for my blessings at the top of that unique house in Gravesend.

My son had a sleep break before the family Christmas dinner was served up. While he was sleeping, I had my time to shower and changed into my Christmas outfit. But that Christmas morning I was cooking our breakfast I was not feeling well, and could not eat the fine food I had prepared for the family, and I felt miserable.

Grandma Anderson would bless our Christmas table. Everyone helped to wash up. I finally went go to sit down. I was still in pain and utterly exhausted. Our family would need to travel back to London at about 10 o'clock or so. The day after Christmas in the UK is 'Boxing Day.' It is not named after the fighting sport, but after a 'Christmas box', an English term for a Christmas present.

Traditionally in England, Boxing Day was a day off of work for servants. They would go home to give Christmas boxes to their own families. That is the day we have here in the UK and Ireland. Another holiday to eat all that food, the leftovers after Christmas. These traditions are steeped in the history and tradition of Victorian era England.

We did not have Christmas trees in this country until Queen Victoria's husband, Prince Albert, introduced them and had them brought over from the continent. Our UK Christmas tree in Trafalgar Square is donated every year by Norway as a token of good will between the two countries.

Holidays were always special to me growing up here in the UK, and now with my own young family growing, the dreadful Christmas and Boxing Day of 1997 was a serious setback. This was the beginning of my battle with MS. As it turned out, 'Boxing Day,' was right; I felt like I had got boxed right in the eyes. It was a *KO* – a straight knockout.

Positive Attitude

Illness is a challenge! Yet, I see it as a blessing in my life. There are many of us around the world with serious diseases. It is up to us as to how we cope with them. I have changed my way of life from a dreadful challenge, to a positive situation. Just by tweaking my diet, getting regular exercise, and disciplining my mind.

Why would you want to harm yourself and beat yourself up? I look at it as these are my cells. I am going to look after myself to the best of my ability. This is not easy in a world of fast foods, and processed foods. But MS, Cancer, Diabetes, Rheumatoid Arthritis, and other chronic diseases are serious illnesses. You have to think about this. This illness sticks to us. It has become a part of us.

You are also in charge of your own positive mental attitude. We *choose* the way we look at things. You have so much power over your own body you would not believe it. Mind truly rules over matter.

Think of when you have accident and you get hurt. Your body automatically starts to heal. We may undergo an operation. Think of how fast our body heals itself from that.

Our minds, spirit, and attitudes affect our bodies. We need to do what we can to stimulate our bodies natural healing processes. Nature is good. Our bodies are good. They are all strong.

The Unique Power of a Woman's Body

As a woman, let me speak to that awesome power we have inherent in our bodies. We have the power to give birth and life to another human being. We then can feed our babies from our own body.

Think of how we have the ability to go through so many changes in our body in pre-birth pregnancy as we carry the baby. We endure much pain but bring forth life. It is truly awesome. The sublime power of women's bodies.

Then there are the hormone changes in our bodies, our periods and menses ebb and flow, to give another chance for life in the body of a woman. There is some conjecture that men feared women in primitive societies, since they bled every month, but did not die. Who knows? But that is power.

Eventually we deal with menopause. Like pregnancy, it can cause weight gain, hot flushes and mood swings. It is a time of transition, of consolidation of strength. Our hard-won life experience matures to wisdom, and our bodies reflect that.

Women's bodies are a storehouse of innate natural wisdom and power. We need to tap into that natural wisdom and power to gain the edge over our mutual enemy of MS.

There are challenges unique to our bodies that we have to deal with, of course. Besides the pain of pregnancy and childbirth, we also have a monthly visitor that men do not have to think about. How do we cope with our hormonal changes with all this?

Menopausal Hot Flushes

Menopause is obviously a challenging time to deal with serious medical conditions. Menopausal mood swings can be managed with a healthy diet.

Some studies have shown that vitamin B6 and Hormone Replacement Therapy (HRT) can protect against osteoporosis and certain cancers. The right foods will give you the right balance with oestrogen, which is in your brain, too. Through just changing our diet a little, we can enhance our body's oestrogen levels. So which foods are high in oestrogen?

Foods that are high in oestrogen include seeds:

Flaxseeds and sesame seeds.

Vegetables that are high in oestrogen are:

Yams, carrots, spouts, kale, celery. Do not forget olives, olive oil, peas and legumes, like pinto beans and chickpeas.

Fruits that are high in oestrogen include:

Apricots, oranges, strawberries, peaches and many dried fruits. Eat them up! They are delicious, good for your overall health, and for regulating the hormone levels in your brain and body. By doing that, you can ride out some of the challenges our awesome bodies sometimes have to endure as women.

You have to admit, eating is not a bad way to deal with such problems.

4: AN UNEXPECTED TESTING

That year ended finally on December 31st, 1997. Once again, I was awarded the honour of being the Top Sales Woman the Automobile Association (AA) for the third year. Kay, my late dear friend, manned the AA stand in Lakeside Shopping Centre in Essex while I tried my best to drive over the Queen Elizabeth Bridge, back to Kent.

I was heading for a medical examination at the Queen Mary Eye Hospital in Sidcup and I was scared witless driving with only the sight of one eye on normal roads. Coming over that crazy long bridge to get my eye exam was a harrowing experience.

'Oh, Shit', I thought. What a silly thing for me to do on my own, driving unaccompanied.

At the hospital, the doctor asked, "Please, could you provide a urine sample,"

"Why?" I replied.

"Because of the radiation. We need to use it for a brain scan. We have to make sure you are not pregnant so that we don't expose the foetus to the radiation," replied the doctor.

"Oh OK, I thought I was here for an eye test, not a pregnancy test."

I took the covered-up urine sample over to the nurse. To my astonishment, she told me that the test came back *positive*.

"Holy Crap!" I replied.

"You're pregnant!" said the doctor, "so we cannot give you an 'MRI' Scan!"

To say that I was shocked is a massive understatement. Of course, there was some more interesting news to follow regarding my eyes.

"Demyelinating inflammation of the optic nerve," was the conclusion of the doctor.

When my mother asked me, "What did the Doctor say?" I tried my best to explain what I understood of all the medical jargon.

"The doctor said it might be Optic Neuritis," I replied.

"What is that?" she asked.

"I really don't know. I have to have an MRI Scan. The blindness could be started by anything – like MS. But all sorts of different things could cause this; certain bacterial infections, Lyme disease, a scratch, or a viral infection, such as mumps measles. To be fair," I said, "it could be a number of things, causing my vision to go."

Mum got back to the topic of MS. "Don't be silly! It could not be MS causing this. That does not run in our family."

Oh how wrong she was.

"The doctor cannot scan me," I told my mum.

"Why not?" she asked.

"Because I am pregnant."

"Pregnant again?" she asked, shocked.

"Yes, Mum,"

"Only you could go to the eye hospital and return being told that you are pregnant!" she said.

"Yes," I replied with a nervous laugh, not wanting her to know how I really felt.

"That could only happen to you!" she said.

I laughed again... nervously.

Later, looking at me through an eye lens, the Doctor said, "It looks very inflamed and swollen."

"Oh, so what does that mean?" I asked.

"It could be the start of optic neuritis, which is your main optic nerve. This can sometimes lead to MS," he replied.

"If this is the cause, an MRI scan can detect any abnormal tissue in the brain, like a brain lesion from an MRI imaging test," the doctor concluded on that rather ominous note.

A possible MS diagnosis. Having MS is where your very own immune system attacks the tissue surrounding the nerve fibres in the brain and Central Nervous System (CNS).

The spinal cord and optic nerve from the back of the eye, each a pair of cranial nerves, transmit impulses to the brain from the retina to the back of the eye. This covering is made of a fatty substance called 'Myelin.' More than half of the people with MS experience this vision problem called 'Optic Neuritis.'

There was so much information swirling around in my mind. I seemed to have gone into a daze. I kind of just switched off.

The Doctor asked, "Are you OK?"

"Pardon?" I replied. "Oh yes. Yes, thank you," I managed to say.

Honestly, I was much more concerned about my pregnancy, to the point where I almost forgot about my eye. I was no longer looking through rose-coloured glasses at my life. This was going to be a real tough ride.

I had only just gone back to work after maternity leave with my son and I was in dispute with the Automobile Association after requesting only part-time hours after my son was born. I needed more time to recover and rest a bit, though that is nearly impossible with a 20-month-old boy.

The dispute was finally settled, thankfully, with full time wages, part-time hours and with reduced sales targets. I had to work just three days a week and could use my company car.

Here I was pregnant again! With baby number two! How I was to explain this news to my boss when he last said, "Number one in sales again this year! No more babies, Maria." Whoops! Nature took its course again.

I could not wait until I told my partner. He would be excited since he eventually wanted a whole football team of kids... However, what we ended up with was two tennis players!

Deep down in my heart, I was scared. I thought I would lose my vision in both eyes permanently. I started to get a slight pain in my other 'good' eye. I later found out, it was stress and worry that was causing that pain. Stress is a root cause of many illnesses.

It was keeping me awake at night for hours – thinking and worrying. Mother used to always say, "Don't sit too close to the TV or you will damage your eyesight!" That was a myth, the Eye Doctor told me. The closer you sit, the better, rather than straining your eyes sitting too far back from the TV. In those days we only had a 9" black and white TV screen.

I saw the ultrasound scan, of my second unborn child. I was about six to seven weeks along in my pregnancy. I would lay awake, planning in my head. I sometimes thought to myself, *what is there for me in the future being blind?*

Tears would roll down the side of my face from both my eyes, around onto the back of my head, and land upon the pillow. Staring up above to the mirror ceiling, hoping not to wake my children's father, I sniffled, quietly, to stop my nose running.

My heart was broken. I was so upset. It was time to come to terms with the loss of the sight in my right eye. It was time to stop feeling sorry for myself. I had a son only 20 months old to take care of. I had to be strong for him.

I was very emotional. It was not like me to cry. Yet, tears just kept flowing like a stream. I have always been a positive person. This was so out of character for me. I have always had a Positive Mental Attitude, but sometimes, life just hits you with the unexpected.

Going blind, having Optic Neuritis, I then realized life had irreversibly changed for me. I also believe God does not give us what we cannot cope with. Everything is for a good reason. MS was meant for me, so as to help others from my own experience in battling with it.

This is all part of my journey – whether I like it or not.

Natural Intelligence of the Body

None of us are ready for an incurable illness. But, our bodies have inbuilt mechanisms to help us heal. Just like when our body reacts when we feel the cold. It is in our body's nature to make us shiver. It will cause itself to shiver so that the power it generates in our body to warm up will create heat. Our bodies have an inbuilt natural intelligence.

You have to have faith that you have this in yourself. That faith will start to heal you alone. It all starts in our minds. This is why, when we are diagnosed with a serious illness, and doctors only give us a limited time to live, we often live right up to the time they tell us. Because we believe them with our thoughts and mind power.

Think of the incredible power of the mind. Think of one person as an example; Professor Stephen Hawking. For so many years, suffering from the debilitating disease he lived with. Physically, emotionally, spiritually and definitely mentally, in every way he contributed to this world. This is the power of the mind. Amazing that he persevered against those odds

Some days I forget I have got Multiple Sclerosis. If I eat well, it is like a domino effect. You start feeling fabulously extraordinarily *well* in your body. Some other days, I feel fatigue, tiredness, and numbness. Yet, each day above ground is a good day – a gift.

I find that I am OK if I am not around too much toxic stress. This will have an effect on your health and wellbeing. This can also happen with any toxic food that I may eat and let enter my body. We need to protect our external environment, and cultivate a healthy inner-environment.

How I Changed

I starting replacing processed foods as they were making me sick. They were giving me migraines, hot sweats, stomach cramps, and constipation. My stool was difficult to pass and very hard. At other times, I would have irritable bowel syndrome. I would feel so dehydrated all the time.

Over the first year of eating fresh as possible organic food, I radically improved. Slowly, I started introducing lots of green vegetables, the greener the better, into my daily diet.

Then came gluten-free grains, like brown rice, quinoa, and millet. These grains are packed with protein, fibre and vitamins. These types of grains satisfy your appetite so you feel full for longer after eating.

I also started cutting out saturated fat altogether from my diet. I started keeping away from dairy products and replacing these things with alternative foods. It is easier to cut out foods when you start replacing them with other tasty foods. I only buy wheat-free, gluten-free bread.

Bread with seeds and nuts is delicious toasted. Eaten dry it has a crunchy texture. They are not all the same in taste. Try different brands until you are satisfied. There are so many more varieties around in all the shops and supermarkets to choose from these days. There are now more health food stores available than ever before.

Weight Loss

Are you the right weight for your height? Try using the Body Mass Index (BMI) as a tool. I find as my weight goes up, then my energy goes down. I find more difficulty in walking, since the additional weight increases the pains in my joints. In my shoulders, ankles, but especially in my knees. MS is a lot harder if you are hauling around extra weight through all that pain.

Blood Sugar is Critically Important

Are there the right levels of all things in your blood count? Do you have high sugar levels and high blood glucose? Sugar has a lot to do with nerve damage. It can affect a loss of hearing, since high blood glucose levels damage the auditory nerves. Excess sugar in your blood will cause your circulatory vessels to narrow. This could restrict the blood supply to your limbs in a disease called Peripheral Arterial Disease (PAD).

These conditions can cause nausea and vomiting. PAD can also cause tingling in your limbs, to the point where you could have difficulty walking. This could ultimately lead to needing an amputation if it progresses further.

High Blood Glucose can cause clots or fatty deposits inside the blood vessels that supply blood to the neck and your brain. Blockage of blood vessels to your brain could cause you to have a stroke. High Blood Glucose can cause all sorts of symptoms from numbness, to the tingling of your feet.

Blockages of any blood vessels to your heart can cause you to have a heart attack. High Blood Glucose can cause damage to your retina which could lead to blindness.

Blockages could cause you another major illness – Diabetes and high blood pressure are both connected with high cholesterol, obesity, fatigue, blurred vision, and headaches.

Whatcha Gonna Do When it Comes for You?

You can help yourself along the way of this journey by eating your way back to good health. Like me, you can stop eating processed foods, and any foods that are packaged, whenever you possibly can.

To be honest, I did not have a choice of having MS. This is an illness that has no cure as of yet. But, it can be stabilized with good food and exercise. You also need a strong level of willpower. We can build that up step by step. We just go slowly like we walk – one simple step at a time.

5: JOURNEY INTO A TUNNEL

Dreading That Damned Test!

I was fortunate since I was already six weeks pregnant when I first was diagnosed with Optic Neuritis. So, the MRI scan could not and would not be done until my pregnancy was done. When my vision finally came back, my thoughts were, h*ow lucky was I?* That would save me from having to return to the hospital!

The MRI scan, if I had been able to go through with it, would have shown, any active brain inflammation. Single or multiple brain lesions may be seen with the MRI, which will light up (enhance) with injection of the contrast material into your system. They inject the dye into your veins.

The MRI would have shown an enlarged optic nerve also, where your visual symptoms usually progress for the first few weeks. Then, after the loss of vision it may start to recover, but not always. Every person's case is unique.

I believe that having good nutrition within my general diet helped with my vision returning. 90% of my sight eventually returned to my right eye. Good nutrition and hydration, avoiding tobacco, and refraining from extreme exercise, which can be overheating during the acute phase of Optic Neuritis. These things were factors in my favour.

But, the actual prognosis, of course, depends on the underlining cause. With most episodes your vision will spontaneously return within two weeks to three months. Thankfully, mine returned to a 90% capacity. With Optic Neuritis you may recover most of your vision within six months from the onset. But again, the underlying cause may have an effect on that.

MRI's

MRI Brain scans have come such a long way. At one time they were like going through a type of tunnel, a tunnel as big as a washing machine drum, on a stretcher – and the noise was like a tumble dryer drum going around your head or your whole body, depending on whether you were having your head or the base of your spine scanned. Nowadays, the MRI scanners are far more sophisticated.

I have had MRI scans in LA. They are very different than those in the UK. Much more modern and larger machines have since made it a less claustrophobic experience.

Never be afraid of any MRI Scans. They are safe, helpful and they may save your life. They can detect so much about the inside of your brain. The brain is our most complex organ in your body. The MRI can detect even the smallest of problems in this sensitive organ.

For my first MRI experience, I had to show up to King's College Hospital in London. I was asked to lie very still as the dye was injected into my veins. Music was playing in the background.

I had a button to press in my hand in case I needed them to stop for any reason. "Just press the button," I was told. I felt comfortable with that. It took about 45 minutes to have an MRI scan.

Though it was weird and a little scary I pushed through that fear. Why? Because, I was not going to let anything or anyone stop me from finding out what was going on inside my own body. I needed to know so I could move on from there.

This was going to be a challenge with my brain tests and the medical insurance. I had not been diagnosed with anything yet. These expensive tests were always ongoing.

Insurance companies are quick enough to insure you and take your monthly premiums and fees. But, they are slow in paying you out. Still, where there is a will there is a way. I had to find out the source of these problems going on inside my own body.

Staying in my top place with my sales career, being pregnant, raising young children, enduring miscarriages in the past, and life in general – I had so much to have to think about. Honestly though, nothing else mattered as long as my precious baby was safe. Now that my daughter had been born I was able to get the MRI procedure.

I finally took the MRI in 1998, after the birth of my precious daughter. Weeks go into months and months into years. When you are a busy working mother, time seems to fly by. Not having much spare time to stop and think about anything other than your children and surviving.

I was suing my employer for a woman's right to go part time. In legal terms this is called having 'standing' to file the lawsuit. After having three previous miscarriages, and devoting so much (successfully) to a company, I needed some more time in my life to take care of my children and my health.

I was not being obnoxious or contentious. These legal actions needed to be done, so that the company would be fair to us working mothers. Ultimately, my case against the company was successful. I was the only part time sales person in the entire sales force.

When you are passionate and have belief in yourself, you can achieve – you will accomplish much. I had to be tough and pragmatic to survive and get me and my children through this difficult time. Come hell or high water, I was going to get us through this.

Five Decades Ago 'Fast Food' Chains Hit the UK

Our diets were not always like this. Something changed that has had devastating effects on the health of people in the 'developed' world of the United States, United Kingdom, and Europe.

It was different when I was growing up in the UK. We always had a vegetable garden. Some of my friends' families would have allotments' a plot of land rented by an individual for growing vegetables, fruits or flowers. Allotments have been going back to the Anglo-Saxon times.

Back as late as the early 1900's, when the land would be handed over to poor people to grow their foods. At the end of the First World War, it was available to everyone. It was a way of assisting returning service men from the front. It was the Land Settlement 1919. Not just for the poor.

We did not have Fast Food Chains back in my era in the 60's. We would have a home-made dinner made from a fresh chicken, which hours before would be running around the garden. Sitting around the table to all eat together, there was no picking and snacking between meal times. Meals were slower and communal for families. Hence, they were healthier.

We could not leave the table until our food was finished. You had to eat what you were given; only having a larder cupboard to keep food cool on a stone shelf.

In 1913 in the States, the first air-cooled refrigeration unit was mounted on top of an icebox. 1923 was the first self-contained 'fridge', but you had to be wealthy to afford a fridge in your home. 'Organic' was the norm in a sense, because people just picked what they were able to grow in their garden. Pesticides had not been made en mass yet.

Back in those days, having hot running water was not the norm. Then, you had to go into the garden and fill the bathtub (which often had ice on it) with kettles of hot water which you had to boil on the gas stove. Those were the poorer days.

We are mighty rich in our new homes, considering the amount of *stuff* we now have and the frequent trips where we go to the charities to donate all that stuff we no longer need. It shows us how much we do not need at the time we wanted to buy it.

Much of the world lives in a poverty that we cannot fathom. No matter how hard it may be for us in the 'First World,' we have a lot of blessings that enhance our life. We also have some not so great things that we need to control, for our own societal health.

Fast Food Nation

The first McDonald's Fast Food joint opened in November 13th, 1974 in South East London, on Woolwich High Street. It was 43 years ago. I was only 10 years old. It was a treat when we would go on the Woolwich Ferry. Afterwards, my Step Dad, 'Paddy', and I would spend time on the 'farm'. (Unfortunately, Stephen 'Paddy,' Gibbons – my stepfather, a very proud, wonderful man, is no longer with us.)

We had some great times in that garden and the backyard with the chickens and other animals. We rose early to go collecting the eggs in the mornings. The rabbits would be running around chasing the cats, dogs, birds, and hamsters. It was like a real farm, with Shetland ponies. They were the *'Good Ole Days,'* when I was only four years old.

I remember helping out on the farm. It was fun and a great learning experience. I learned to put the potatoes into the soil once they started growing roots. I learned how to go about planting the carrots. Planting the Runner Beans, which would grow to climb up the trellis like in *Jack and the Beanstalk*.

We planted spring onions and garlic. We planted basil, mint and thyme. We planted a bay tree. We even had strawberry plants and grew fresh tomatoes. With the Shetland pony, we had to save the manure. to use it in our garden (It is fine if you are a vegan – you just wash the vegetables and fruit before eating). We would use it on our front lawn too.

We were hardly ever sick, eating like that as kids. Actually, I do not ever recall seeing a doctor during that whole time. This was before so many of us in the UK got used to the American fast food chains. We thought we were in for a real treat to get what the Yanks across the pond had.

In 1965 was when the first Kentucky Fried Chicken opened its doors to the public in the UK It was the American's first Fast Food chain here in the UK, predating its rivals – McDonald's, Burger King, and Pizza Hut by almost a decade.

Truth be told, since the fast food industry hit our country, illness have risen *much* higher. We have tripled our rates of obesity and diabetes, along with a host of neurological illness. Illnesses like MS.

This may be one of the key reasons why MS is more prominent in western developed countries than in the world's developing nations. This is one of the mysteries I was determined to unravel. Where did MS come from, and why did it afflict me? And more importantly, what can I do now that I have it – to fight it.

Medical Detective

I wanted to know, 'why?' My detective work led me to this conclusion for all sorts of reasons. I do not know the specific reason(s) I got MS but I knew I had to fight it. Honestly, the prescribed medications scared me. Some MS patients were afflicted with the dreadful side effects possible in some of the medications.

Some had to be injecting themselves with medications, many on a regular basis. Or, they had to rely on other people to do the injections for them. They took the medications to keep their independence but so many lost it through that path. They just wanted to stay as independent as long as they could.

One of those most frustrating aspects of this journey for us is how long it can take for us to get a clear diagnosis. The endless waiting for insurance approvals, waiting for tests, differing (and often conflicting) medical opinions, etc. But it is part of the journey we need to go on since the earlier this disease is caught, the better.

Early Diagnosis is Critically Important

Early diagnosis is a key factor. The longer you do not know what is wrong with you, the worse for you. An illness could be ticking away like a time bomb waiting to go off inside your body and brain. Or, it may be there just waiting for the next relapse.

Although there is no single finding or test that can *definitively* tell you if you have MS, doctors can use a combination of tests and symptoms to diagnose MS. Thankfully, the technology is getting better.

For example, your doctor will likely perform a neurological exam, an MRI, evoked potentials, and a spinal fluid analysis. They will also want an extensive medical history report from you. These tests and reports will help them to find evidence of damage in at least two different areas of the central nervous system at different points in time and to rule out any other diagnoses. It is a process of elimination, just like when the mechanic works on your car.

When you take that into an account and the doctors would like to start you on 'treatment', ask yourself where will *that go* if there is no 'cure'? When are you asked about your life style? Pretty much never. You need to connect the dots. The medical industry does not have the capacity to delve into your life and habits to see what has been going on in there. Only you can do that.

Maybe you are a heavy smoker, drinker, or perhaps even heading towards being a working alcoholic, an addict, or taking all sorts of drugs (prescriptions or street). Would not those lifestyle factors play a part in it? Of course!

I am not insinuating that MS suffers are drug addicts. I am just saying that the things people do in their life end up manifesting in their bodies. Something caused it. Probably something we engaged in. So, we can 'un-engage' in some things that possibly got us sick.

The argument in my mind was this:

If the above poor lifestyle choices and poor food choices can make you sick, then stopping them and eating healthy should make you feel better. It is really that simple.

If Fast Food and junk food can make you sick (and it will), then 'slow healthy' food can heal you. That makes logical sense, does it not? Slow down with slow healthy food. If we lived in that way at the beginning, then perhaps some of us would not have been stricken with MS.

That is why I started using only organic fresh foods to cook with and dine on. I do it both for the health benefits I have received, *and* for their great taste! Good foods can only do you good.

We can start by staying away from saturated fats, dairy products, wheat, gluten, and all processed foods (especially those made with corn syrup). This crap will cause fat to build up around your heart, making your heart work harder just to get the blood through.

Excessive fat is a major strain on your organs. Excess weight makes you heavy, so it is more difficult to move around. When we are sitting too long in one place, is not good for your health. Have you heard the saying, 'Sitting is the new smoking'?

Breaking Free

We are not 'cured' for as we know there is no cure for MS. We simply overcome. We do this through behaviours that help us in that path of 'overcoming.' That is pretty simple. Is this simple approach worth a try out? The worst that can happen is you will feel better.

This is a marathon, and not a sprint. *'I have always been healthy, so why did I get this?'* I asked myself often. Because we are only human. We are not perfect and we do the best we can with what God gives us.

You cannot beat yourself up. Taking responsibility for our health is the only way out of the hole. I know this now. This worked for me. It has been very liberating, to find myself in control of what I choose to eat.

I *do know* how hard it is to break poor eating habits. But, it really is possible. When it involves your health, anything is possible if you focus on what you desire. Diet along with exercise impacts brain and CNS health. Together they will help to prevent manifestation of MS symptoms.

6: ALL WORK & NO PLAY

Life throws curve balls at us we often do not want, and seldom expect. We set up our plans. But, our plans often have other plans for us.

My partner and I had to rush to the hospital on May 5th of 1995. We were just moving into a house together. I so was excited for our new future. Then it came.

I started to have stomach cramps and I was four months pregnant so we rushed to get things checked out at the hospital. Again, I had miscarried. An awful replay of losing twins in 1990. It broke my heart. I was totally devastated.

So, I focused all my energy into work. Work became my way to take the sorrow and pain away. I became one of the most successful top sales women in England. I set my mind to that, even though the field I ended up working in was completely dominated by men.

It's A Man's World?

High wage paid jobs were for men in 1980's. Only four women were employed at my company at the time I was hired. I ended up driving up to 30,000 miles a year around the entire country for work attending meetings and conferences. And making sales.

This became tough on my relationship with my partner. Truly, we were like the proverbial 'ships passing in the night', as I passed up and down the motorways of the UK, I was working a lot and he was working a lot too. We did not have much time for one another.

Long before our children were born, my partner and I would drive from Kent to London. I would drop him off sometimes at his mother's home in London, where he had parked his work van. We were busy bees; trying to get ahead and get set.

I never paid for fuel, though it would have made sense with my fuel card. Those days it put your mileage up, which brought your tax down in your wages. There was always a logical method to my madness. Then I would carry on my journey to work around the clock. Making sales, making meetings, making it rain.

My partner and I shared the same dream. To invest in property together. 'United we stand and divided we fall'. For both our children, down to this day, we still agree on investment in property.

For our children's future inheritance, we both worked so hard for over 30 years. Our children are our future. We always kept that in mind. Our children are our future literally. They will choose our nursing home in years to come, so be nice to them!

Communication is Key

It is all about giving and sharing together. Equally, *a problem shared, is a problem halved,* goes the saying. That *'in sickness and in health'* stuff means *really talking* together. Communication is the key. Hiding away relationship problems (any problems in fact) does not cut it.

As an adult, a parent is being irresponsible if they do not show a sense of responsibility to their home life. Like with our illness, we feel better talking about problems and addressing them. It reminds us that us we are not alone. You can become very lonely and isolated struggling with MS. You have to communicate with loved ones and family. It is vital in getting you through the challenges of MS.

Technology Can Intrude on Your Family Time

I wonder if families are not becoming even more separated nowadays? So many people have addictions to technology. Technology these days makes people very unsociable because they let it rule their life.

It is like working from home in the middle of your living room. How does a wife feel when 'work' is going on all the time in front of her? Or, even having the TV on and not listening to your husband? Or, a friend or two who is round and you are on the smartphone. Or, using that smartphone to keep the children quiet? It is very alienating and isolating.

All this will contribute to health issues sooner or later – both mental health and physical health. Having an office away from home is healthier if possible. You can socialize with others there, then leave your 'home time' as the time to really be with people in 3D.

Having MS, it is better to keep mobile and moving anyway. As an MS sufferer, if you are still able to work, keep working and moving if you can. Mobility is a key to helping us.

Movement keeps your joints from seizing up. You never know how long you will be mobile for. You never know what you have got until you do not have it anymore. Then your miss it.

Let's not take advantage, or take for granted those people who are in our lives, especially, as we struggle through this disease. All relationships are really temporary; either through leaving, distance, or death. Let's treasure the time we have with our partners, children, grandchildren, friends, and colleagues.

Career Achievements

With my sales job for the motoring clubs, I loved working the boot fairs, garage sales, malls, festivals, and especially working outdoors. I loved my work because I love helping others.

This was before cell phones. The elderly, or single women could get trapped out at night, or in awful weather, and not have a way to get help when their vehicle broke down on the road, or if their tyre blew.

When they purchased what I sold, it was like getting some really important insurance (road insurance) that could help keep them safe. I respected what I sold and how it actually helped many people to have safer lives.

Back when I became the Top Sales Woman in the history of the Automobile Association, it was a 'man's job' in the late 1980's. After then, women began doing the so-called *men's* jobs.

Just four sales women on the road for AA back at that time. Trying to sell membership plans for road insurance and breakdown assistance. We worked hard in extreme weather conditions. We did not have many indoor shopping centres then, like we do today.

I remember working when the hurricane force winds hit the UK on the night of 15th -16th October 1987. There were high winds of 134 mph. This in the island of England! It was the worst storm ever in 300 years, claiming 22 human lives in three hours.

Working in the High Street, trying to keep out of the wind and rain. Selling memberships like hotcakes to keep your job with a company car. Working fifty weekends a year as it was in our contract. It was quite draining at times. We only have a limited amount of life energy.

I finally purchased another property later at the age of 35. I've been a 'landlady' for a decade. It was a huge responsibility. Having three cell phones; one for my work, one for my property management, and a private phone.

I finally sold all the properties in 2012 when I moved to Los Angeles. Hard work pays. The enjoyment is the achievement you receive and feel from hard work. I instilled this work ethic into our children. I pinch myself some days to believe this is not a dream.

I worked hard for the Automobile Association which had been trading since 1905. The Royal Automobile Club has been going since 1897. Having worked for both companies at different times, I learned the inside and outs of the business and focused on success.

I was their top saleswoman for a few years. Being the first woman to achieve those sales targets made me feel good, apart from the monetary reward.

Top Awards in sales (while pregnant four times!) in selling membership and sales of Roadside Assistance Plans. I am proud to say I was also top at selling legal insurance, and top at selling company credit cards.

Always working the Kent County shows. I worked the Kent area of England for 20 years. I am proud to say I was the top sales woman at all time in the County shows. I worked hard all over that island!

I was successful in signing thousands of new members every year in all kinds of crazy UK weather; rain, snow and sun. I met a lot of interesting people in the streets of London, Kent, and all over England. I enjoyed the work a lot. I enjoyed the people.

You can accomplish anything you put your mind to. Never look down on anyone in life is my motto. When you're on the way up to the top of your career, we never know what will come, you may need somebody one day on the way down. The nerdy guy in the mail room today may be the C.E.O one day. I treat everyone with respect. That was a key to my sales success.

True Success

Always believe in yourself, even when you feel like giving up. I strive to lead by pure example, hard work, modesty and discipline. This led to my success. I was happy with my career. It was never about the money for me. It was purely about the success of the achievements.

Through all my life's ups and downs, I have learned that there are three important things in your life: Time, Health, and Energy. The truth is this – what you put out you get back tenfold. I put out a lot.

Money is important in order to live. Money is important when you are sick, especially with a serious chronic disease. But would it not make more sense to avoid getting sick and staying healthy? That would be better than having the money to pay for treatments *after* you lose your health.

No one knows what your future holds. It is always important to have critical heath care coverage to weather emergencies. Some chronic diseases where you just cannot work due to a disability, but the disability is not obvious. Not all disabilities are visible.

In all these things we must remember life is often like the weather. Not all storms come to disrupt your life. Some just come along to clear your path.

You are all unique in your journey. There is no comparison with others. Just like the sun and the moon. You will shine when it is your time in life. Who knows if that is not the case with all this illness we have to deal with?

The bottom line is this: It not about how big your house is, or how big your bank account is, or how new your car is. We all will have the same size grave in the end. You are taking nothing with you.

Positive Attitudes Can Heal

You are in charge of your own life. Getting older, I realize how important our attitude is on the quality of our life. We are all in charge of our own attitudes and destiny. We can choose to have faith and hope.

It has been said that a quarter of things '*just happen*' to you in your life. What is most important is the three quarters that is left – which is how we can react. That part is under our control.

From all of the many intelligent people I know, there are a few who live mostly in the past. This makes them rather foolish, in spite of their intellectual gifts. Living in the past cannot help them heal. There is no future there in your past. The past has gone; the future is not here yet. All we have is right *now*. What are we doing with that 'precious now'?

Having a positive mental attitude helped me heal. Our attitude is our own issue to fix. Just like nobody can count another person's money in life. It is on us. You are an amazing, unique and special individual – who happens to have an illness. You are so much more than your illness. Always remember this. You are not your illness!

Integration

We always have the best intentions. Reality does not care about our intentions. Nothing and no one does. Changes happen due only to *actions*. It is not what we *say*, it is what we *do* that makes an impact. The time has come to choose which of these healthy lifestyle patterns you are going to integrate first. Understand what your deepest motivation for change and health is. Then commit. Action always takes place *now*, not tomorrow. Act as if your life hangs on it. For in reality, it may.

7: AIM HIGH IN THE SKY

What Are You Living For?

When your alarm clock goes off in the morning, do you dread waking up? Then you might as well go straight back to sleep, or quit the job you're doing. If it is a career you do not like waking up to, then you are in the wrong job. If it is the gym you do not like, you're at the wrong gym. Why just go through the motions of living?

In my sales career, I loved my job. It gave me great personal satisfaction to achieve success in helping people. I felt proud just knowing that on their journey they were covered. They would be safe with their loved ones, family and children not stranded on a motorway, or ripped off by unknown towing company. That gave me a sense of purpose in my three decades of working hard and successfully in that field.

Now, finally my dreams came true through faith and hard work. My dream was to be mortgage free at the age of fifty. Everyone needs a dream. Everyone needs a focus. Aim for the moon – you could get to the stars. Reach and aim high, whatever your dreams may be.

I am enjoying this time. I am enjoying the beauty of the life of the universe around us. Enjoy this abundance that surrounds us. We can enjoy it more fully with balance:

'It is not what you have, it is what you give that counts'.

I *could* retire. It is my time now. I cannot work at a job due to my illness, but I am going to make it work! Now, my work is researching all the best foods for our immune system to restore energy and health. I have experimented with these approaches of healthy eating and exercise. They work. So my 'work' now is to share this good news.

'Good health is our true wealth', so the saying goes. This is not just a trite phrase. It is profoundly true. MS (or any chronic illness) can be controlled and defeated, if not officially 'cured'. We can often mitigate the disease's symptoms. With healthier eating habits many illnesses have been reversed.

The wisdom of this challenge with MS (or any other illness) is to channel the energy of this experience to become who you really are. Your true identity. Be smart! We are intelligent human beings; bright, alert, insightful, perceptive and keen. Let us apply our minds and spirits to the task of healing and recuperating.

For *you*, and *you only*, can take control of your healing.

True Confessions

When I got the dreaded news of having incurable Multiple Sclerosis, to be honest, my heart hit rock bottom. I felt my bubble had burst. My life, I felt, had *ended*.

"The Doctors must be wrong!" my Mother had said, "It is not in our family history!" I am too young, too healthy, too busy with life to deal with this! My mind had these and many more angry, denying thoughts swirling through my mind. And, *I stayed in denial for a long, long time afterwards*.

I knew I had to find out the truth about this dreaded illness that had afflicted me. This illness that has no known cure. I knew I needed to find a way of coping – without using prescribed medication. My body was too sensitive for those and I knew I would have bad reactions. I always did.

Then, I learned that being *stress free* and keeping a *positive mindset* could help stabilize my illness. This was like some light that I saw through a key hole, so I opened the door. It opened up a new life for me.

This all starts within your mind. Being determined (or stubborn!) will help you. You will have *knock-backs* for sure. That is life. For everyone, life has its ups and downs. Just like the waves of the ocean.

By having the motivation to believe you can get stronger every day – you will succeed. Just through changing your eating habits – slowly over time (the same way the illness came on). Victory is well within your reach.

My dream for this book is that it may be like a pebble thrown into the ocean. It splashes! Then the ripples of water reach out around the world in different languages to different people. People in hospitals, in a hospice, in medical centres, people in their homes. People everywhere that can benefit from reading and applying it.

I want this book to help as many human beings as possible. So, I am sharing this way of life which has helped me heal – even down to healing the cells of the lesions in my brain. I have worked hard through all these approaches. I want to share what has worked with you.

I am Not Your Doctor

Only a Doctor can give you advice – or your consultant or MS nurse. I am not those. I am not giving you advice, since I cannot do that. I am just giving you *my own experiences.* I am merely sharing my achievements from the exercise and natural diet approach I used.

What worked for me might just work for you. So, give it a try. You have nothing to lose (apart from a few pounds). Most of us can stand to lose a little weight, to gain some more mobility, or even just to grow a smile again on our face.

If I can help even just a few of my readers, then my dreams will have come true. Then I have manifested my dream through positivity. My hope is that *you have hope* in your life. My happiness is in seeing that everyone who crosses my path heals a bit – both mentally and physically.

Gaining hope and confidence will give you a better life with MS. You are responsible for your own health so have a specific vision. Focus on your own feelings – in your emotions and your physical body. Everything happens by the Spirit in our body. Your thoughts and attitudes are what will bring your harmony.

My Cells and Me – Osteoporosis

I am now much better after caring for my *individual cells*, because they are all a part of me. I have had to learn this over the years living with MS and Osteoporosis. Both diseases have no cure, yet, through the principles I share in this book, I have reversed my Osteoporosis.

Osteoporosis is a common condition among people with MS. They seem to go hand in hand. The bones in your body become very brittle and weak.

A research article from Norway argued that Multiple Sclerosis is a cause of Secondary Osteoporosis, leading to a host of other medical complications. Bone mineral density decreases when an individual's MS disability increases.

Osteoporosis is a progressive condition that causes your bones to become brittle. Having MS increases your risk for lower bone density. This would put you at a higher risk of a bone fracture. This is why I eat good nutritious food and engage regularly in exercise.

It was not easy living with Osteoporosis in Los Angeles in 2014. My bone scan had indicated to the doctors that I needed to start taking 70 milligrams of Alendronic Acid. I have one tablet a week (always on a Sunday) with a pint of water. But on the down side, you do need to be near a toilet when it's been taken! It takes around an hour before I can eat or drink anything else after taking those meds.

Osteoporosis can also can cause the very painful experience of *Sciatica*. This is a condition where the primary spinal nerve gets irritated or pinched. Take my word for it – it is no fun.

The Sciatic Nerve

The sciatic nerve is the largest and longest spinal nerve in the human body. It extends from the lumbar and sacral plexuses in the lower back. The sciatic nerve runs through the buttocks and into the thighs. It delivers nerve signals to and from the muscles and skin of the thighs, lower legs and feet.

Sciatica is very painful. The causes can be numerous, but it is often associated with Osteoporosis. I learned from my medical consultant in Los Angeles how to stop the pain:

Lift your left leg and place your right ankle on top of your left knee. Then hold the position for a moment. This will help stretch your tiny piriformis muscles. Clasp both hands behind your thigh locking your fingers. This sometimes becomes inflamed and then presses against the sciatic nerve, causing you pain.

They also shared this jewel of a pain-relieving exercise:

Try the 'Sitting Pigeon' yoga pose. You sit on the floor with your legs stretched out straight in front of you. Bend your right leg, by putting your right ankle on top of your left knee. Lean forward and allow your upper body to reach toward your thigh. Hold that for about 20 to 30 seconds. This will stretch your glutes and lower back. Then repeat on the other side. Then do the same exercise with your other leg by rotating your hips.

I loved this pose. It literally stopped my pain. It works.

Environmental Hazards

You could say pollution from carbon fuels and diesel across the UK, to the smog in Los Angeles are further health hazards for us. Especially those of us with auto-immune disorders, like MS. Our 'autos' may be triggering our 'auto'-immune systems to crash.

The carbon fumes do have a lot to do with our inner bodies and how they function. The sooner you can get out of that car from the hustle and bustle in traffic jams the better for your health.

Whether it is the 405 Freeway in LA or the M25 Motorway in the UK, none of it is good for those of us struggling with MS. We have to get out and smell the fresh air, the smell of trees in the London Parks, or the walks in Kent, 'the Garden of England'. If you are in LA, head to the beach or mountains every time you can, can get a positive O2 fix. Clean air is powerfully healing. It increases the oxygenation of our cells and tissues.

When I was living in LA, I would hit Manhattan Beach, Hermosa Beach, Redondo Beach and Santa Monica Beach. I would often go down to Venice or Malibu Beach. Listen to the sound of the ocean to rock to peace your restless soul. Then smell of the salty sea air. Let it clean your lungs and internal organs. The best and healthiest things we can do for ourselves are truly free. Breathing is free.

Healing Naturally is, Well, Natural

It cannot be too difficult or overly technical to heal naturally if we focus on healing with simple recipes, herbs, and spices blended together. These simple steps can help to heal joint pain and bring our bodies into a state of equilibrium.

When Inflammation occurs chemicals from your body's white blood cells are released into your circulatory system and into the affected tissues. It is our bodies way to protect us from foreign substances and intruders.

This release of these chemicals increases the blood flow to the area of injury or infection. This results in redness and warmth in the area. The right combination of naturally grown organic products, spices, and herbs can reduce this inflammation. Sometimes quite significantly.

Sharing the specifics of some of these natural combinations of and recipes of how to use these anti-inflammatory foods, herbs, and spices will be what we are turning to soon. Not only will I share the specific ones to use, I will share a bit on how they work.

Remember how I shared that I was a professional chef and baker for many years and that is one of my main passions? Well you are in for a treat. I wish I could come into each of your homes, and show you just how easy it is to prepare excellent tasting, satisfying, delicious natural food preparations, meals and snacks. Your mouth would water seeing and smelling it!

8: EATING YOUR WAY TO HEALTH

My Change to Becoming a Pescatarian

I eat so much fish that I feel like I will be growing fish gills soon! I now can swim up and back in that pool as fast as a torpedo being fired from a submarine having so much energy. Am I turning into a fish? Ha! Sometimes I wonder, since they say, 'you are what you eat', I do swim much faster than I used to.

With an MS diagnosis having fish in your diet is *a must* to help repair the damaged brain and nerve cells. For everyone, but especially for us, *food matters*. Food makes such a difference to a successful healing process.

It will take some time to change the eating habits of a lifetime. It has taken me five years (and still growing and learning). There is that old saying I joked about above – 'We are what we eat.' and, 'A touch on your lips, is a lifetime on your hips.' I could not agree more with these old proverbs.

Patience is a virtue and it is said that it comes to those who wait. But, it needs to hurry up! I am not always that virtuous. I struggle for patience just like everyone. The dietary changes I have integrated into my life have helped me maintain better equilibrium and to have more patience.

These simple lifestyle changes have *radically* helped with my aches and pains in my back, my knee joints and the inflammation so common with MS.

I am also basically now pretty much free of migraine headaches through my changed diet. I stopped feeling weak and tired. I have more energy – and them some!

Ages 20 to 50 There *is* deterioration in our bodies – Not from our age, but rather how we choose to live

Take a look how you have lived over the past 20 years. A fraction of your life already has gone by. Ultimately, ageing is just a belief system, since your body renews and transforms its cells from *old* to *new* all the time. Technically, every seven years we have completely new cells from what we had seven years prior.

By what I choose to eat – my body age is 15 years younger than what my Driver's License says it is. This is not about *the number* of the years. It has to do with my lifestyle; what I choose to eat, drink and if I do my regular exercise.

Positive, healthy choices and actions are restorative but negative ones are very damaging to our body and soul. Try to stop focusing on how *stressed* you are and remember how *blessed* you are! The mind, spirit and the body act as one unit. We need to truly know that and work that fact to heal.

Practice deep *acceptance* and *forgiveness* to heal your hurts, disappointments, resentments, and residual anger from the past. Any jealously is the simply the inability to share in another person's joy or happiness, so you are cutting yourself off from blessings. Always remember, we have bigger hearts than that.

Life is far too short to be at war within oneself. Stop tormenting yourself with negative, angry, unproductive thinking. It is said that not forgiving someone or something is like taking a poison and expecting someone else to die from it. In reality, we die from it.

True happiness and true wealth is the ability to experience and appreciate each living moment for everything it is worth. It is not what *happens to you* in your life, but how you *respond* to what happens that really counts in the end.

Always focus on counting God's blessings, while others are adding up and calculating all their troubles in life. Having a *Positive Mental Attitude* affects how we do *everything*; how we digest, how we sleep, how we rest, how fast we heal, and how happy we are.

Keep laughing! It is the cheapest medicine. When you keep laughing about the life you're living you will end up with a life worth smiling about. You will make those around you happier too.

Diets – Do They Really Work?

Fad diets will not send you in a straight line forward, but instead will 'yo-yo' your body back and forward throughout your life. I believe that if you have MS, you need to get serious about what you eat, not follow some silly fad diet. *Transformation* is not a temporary change. Be about changing your eating habits – for good.

I have had to do this through my own struggle with this illness. So start this journey like you truly mean to go on to a new, more energetic, healthier you. This is a real deadly and debilitating illness, so let's get serious about transforming our patterns of eating.

These first steps may seem scary or insurmountable. Breaking old habits is tough. Just remember, we are not really *breaking* anything! We are *introducing* something new and tasty as a replacement.

You like trying new food? Who does not? Cultivate that attitude in your mind. Then your tongue, stomach and eating habits will quickly catch up. We are not *depriving* ourselves, we are *enlivening* ourselves with richer, tastier, healthier foods.

For example, you will notice that after three weeks of cutting out processed sugar items from your diet that your taste buds will change. Then, if you take in processed sugar again, it will taste *too* sweet. To the point where it is a bit gross.

Traditional diets and 'fad' diets are not all they are cracked up to be for our health. Many so-called 'low fat' foods contain a load of other bad sugars, chemicals, carbohydrates and unhealthy fats – which are hidden.

Good natural fats will build up your joint linings, tendons, brain and nerve cells, reproductive organs, and even muscles. Eating naturally and healthily is just like a doing a workout at the gym. The more you work your muscles, the stronger they will get. This regularity of habit is what will make you stronger – without sacrificing anything in taste or fullness.

There is a saying, 'If you do not use it, you will lose it' so let your taste buds *evolve* and get stronger, more discerning. Have good fats, proteins, and natural fruit sugars in moderation to help repair your cells damaged from MS.

You only have to look at body builders to see how they feed their muscles to become fit and strong for competitions. You too, are in a competition, the reward being freedom from the symptoms of MS. Take you nutrition seriously Champ!

These tips and recipes in the back of this book will not only be of help for MS patients. They are solid advice for everyone's body. The caregivers we have in our life will suffer and run out of steam if they do not eat right. *We all* need to feed our bodies and brains with the good natural nutrition that our bodies need and crave.

'Superfoods' – For a Super You

What is a 'Superfood?' Superfoods are natural foods, mostly plant-based (but, some meats and diary) that are profoundly *nutritionally dense*. Superfoods are considered to have some healing proprieties since they are so rich in nutrition. A little of them goes a long way.

Wheatgrass is my 'go to' Superfood. I swear by it. It reduces my tiredness and fatigue. It is full of calcium, Vitamin E, high in iron and protein. I only add ½ a teaspoon to my yoghurt or healthy juice. Like I said, a little goes a long way.

Another Superfood I recommend is Spirulina. What is Spirulina? It is a form of 'cyanobacteria' which is a family of single-celled microbes, often referred to as 'blue-green algae.' Just like plants, cyanobacteria produce energy from sunlight via photosynthesis. Spirulina are single-cell organisms that can live in both fresh and salt water.

The ancient Aztecs used to eat Spirulina for energy. In modern times, even NASA recommended it as a nutritionally dense 'space food' that astronauts can take on extended trips into long missions into outer space.

Spirulina has very high levels of protein which is great, especially if you do not eat meat or are a vegan. Spirulina has many different B vitamins. You need these especially with MS to support your immune system. Is also high in magnesium and iron.

Spirulina is anti-inflammatory and it raises the 'good' cholesterol and reduces the bad cholesterol. It is helpful for high blood pressure and anaemia. Some researchers suggest it may be good for cancer patients.

I only add half a teaspoon to my yoghurt, or healthy juice every morning before my exercise workouts. It is very energizing eating Superfoods which come from organic fresh ingredients.

I try to incorporate as many Superfoods into my diet as possible. Superfoods help detox my inner body gently. I love feeling better while the food I eat cleans my system, but tastes great! What an easy and delicious way to get healthier.

I use all-natural ingredients in my own recipes I have created. I do not have much extra time in my schedule, so I created recipes that you can prepare quickly and easily – from vegetarian to vegan recipes.

I do have a few recipes for the meat-eaters too! From Jamaican curry goat, to ackee and salt fish that I learned from my late mother-in-law, the Grandma to my children. These recipes will be included in my next book.

No More Excuses

One of the excuses people use to justify persisting in eating unhealthy food is that, 'good food is expensive.' If you think you cannot afford to eat well, rethink that mentality – because you also cannot afford to be sick! Are you independently wealthy and do not have to work? Congratulations, but most folks need to be able to work.

Getting seriously sick will put you *way back* with your money situation, both from what you have to pay out, and what you can no longer earn from working due to illness.

It basically boils down to this: *Pay now or pay later.*

Good Food Can Benefit Your Moods

Good healthy food will help with your mood swings; the high and lows, and even depression. I truly believe these mental states have a lot to do with our diet. There are plenty of studies that show that.

Even with our children's behaviour, consider the role of their diet. I changed my son and daughter's diet. The difference it made to their behaviour while growing up was immense! When I changed their foods they were much more stable and even-keeled as children.

It was a phenomenal help to their concentration and their behaviour at school. They were both like different children. I never heard of Attention Deficit Hyperactivity Disorder (ADHD) back when I was a kid at school. I was just naughty, or maybe I did have it? Who knows? I just know that we are (and act) as we eat – we and our children.

Let's Get to It – Healthy Fats and The Brain

You are free to follow what I have been doing. If it feels good and positive, then you are heading in the right direction. This path does work and I am living-proof it is still working.

Although we are all different, this approach to mitigating the symptoms of MS may also work wonders for you, so join me now. No more excuses like, 'next week, next month, etc.' We, as people with MS, cannot afford that luxury of procrastination. We have this now. We need to deal with it now.

You do need to examine in detail how much processed, fast foods, 'take away' foods, and junk foods you consume. Then break it down in a journal or pad all the components of what you eat, how much, and when. Do it for a week.

Take a look at your food cupboard. Ideally, they should be pretty empty. Tins, cans, processed foods generally are not good for us. Let's instead, have the fridge full of fresh, ready to eat organic fruit and vegetables to snack on.

For example, avocado (yum, full of good fat!). Avocado is one of best foods you can consume for the health of the brain. I cut my avocado in half, remove the stone, skin it, then freeze the half I am not using. Then you can remove it from freezer when you want more. It takes about 30 minutes to thaw. If you slice it as its half thawed you can eat it with a salad. I like mine not too thawed out – to the point where it's a bit mashed.

Blueberries, beets and broccoli – The 3 B's. Eat lots of celery, coconut oil and occasionally some dark (low sugar) chocolate. The most effective Omega-3 fats occur naturally in oily fish, in the form of EPA and DHA.

There are also good plant sources for healthy fats. These include linseed, flaxseed, pumpkin seeds, walnuts and their oils. Theses fats are very important for healthy brain function, for your heart, your joints, and overall well-being.

Just like an automobile needs oils to function, your body needs clean, healthy oils for internal lubrication – for all the pistons (nerves) to 'fire.' These healthy fats are our body's internal lubrication. We are 'changing our oil' in a sense, every time we consume healthy fats.

Eating good fats not *only* boosts your strength. The proper fats and nutrients in your food are also excellent fuel for your brain. In the USA, researchers have discovered that a few walnuts daily, over time, helps makes you calm. They are also a good source of vitamins.

Our brain needs fuel food. Though the brain makes up only 2% of our body weight, it uses up 20% of our entire body's energy. We need to feed it the right foods if we are going to think right.

Whatever you choose to bite, chew, and swallow has a profound effect on the organs and their systems in your body. You do have a choice for every bite of food you eat. It will either deplete or nourish your brain. Who wants to starve their brain?

By consuming unhealthy foods, like sugars, trans fats, etc., these can really make your brain feel fuzzy and foggy. You can also start to feel depressed and often anxious. Our moods are very connected to our diets and what passes our lips.

If Bad Foods Can Contribute to Illness – Then The Reverse Should Also Be True

Our body's illness must be able to be reversed and heal – if you feed that's what it needs. Re-train your tongue to crave healthy food. It is natural for you to love natural food. It is in our DNA. Follow that line back to what your ancient ancestors ate that gave them strength and stamina. You can heal from food without the side effects of prescribed medication.

Being Vegan

I tried being a raw vegan for a month. To be honest, it can be a very boring life. It does depend on the illness you have as to how much you want to detoxify your body. Raw vegan is pretty hard core for setting up a full deep body detox.

By going on a raw vegan detox, I noticed all the wind disappeared from my stomach – the swelling, discomfort, pain etc. It all was going down from making that dietary change.

The doctor thought I was heading for Irritable Bowel Syndrome (IBS). When I ate processed foods, I would have stomach cramps and diarrhoea. (I know, TMI – Too Much Information!).

The effects seemed almost like I had some kind of food poisoning.

I had experienced actual food poisoning twice before by eating prawns in the hot weather. You can also get this from contact with another person, or from contaminated water. It is often the contaminated water left on produce that makes people sick in restaurants.

Having your stool run away from you – you shit like a goose. I know, TMI again! I was semi-back to normal, going to the toilet ('number 2s') up to three times a day after I had turned vegan.

In a vegan diet you do eat a lot of fibre which of course is great for our systems. It is when you have eaten meat that the worst problems occur. Meat stays in your digestive system for a *longggg* time, putting more strain on your whole system. The length of time it is being digested is what builds up the toxins that go into our bloodstream.

Time to Make A Change – To What?

Consider just becoming a 'flexitarian' to start. Be flexible, but begin to gradually introduce some of these healthier things to eat. It takes time, but just start to do it. You will be shocked by how tasty the food is, how much better you can feel in a rather short time. It will quickly become addictive to eat well.

Just find replacements – 'like for like' foods. That way you are not feeling like you are missing out on anything. Keep yourself interested and experimenting. Your taste buds will change over time. And, so will your health.

They say Rome was not built in a day. We did not get sick in one day either, it took a lot of decisions over time that got us to where we are. We just have to work our way back, undoing the bad things we have previously been doing, replacing them with good habits, and being patient with ourselves.

This is really about just loving yourself. Do you love yourself? Ask yourself that question. If not, why not? Work through that. If so, then let that truth affect your every decision on how you treat your unique and precious body. God gave each of us only one – Let's treat it as the precious gift it is. We do that through one small choice at a time.

9: FALLING FORWARD INTO NEW LIFE

My Moves Across the Pond

Did I really want to stay in California just being sick? Not really. We moved five times in three years. That was stressful and tiring in and of itself. But I went there to live with my new husband and to see if I could heal better there in the States.

Eventually, I knew I needed to be home – in a country where you are looked after if need be, like England. To be honest, there is no place like home. I was missing it, though there were parts of living in the States that I loved.

Having MS is no joke. I felt my energy levels take a drop to a new low level. California was getting hotter year by year. With the heat and my condition, it knocked me sideways — literally.

Learning to Fall Before Learning to Fly

I had started falling regularly. We had gone to LA to go to some speciality medical clinics that focused on MS patients. But I was having a rough time of it. These incidents of falling became more frequent, and frankly I was scared.

Holding onto my husband's strong arm, my confidence fell away farther the more times I fell. I was getting scared and feeling vulnerable. Falling regularly and unpredictably is very disorienting. Basically, it sucks.

It happened in the cinema a couple of times in Manhattan Beach in Southern California. When I fell and went down, my coffee went down onto my hand and burnt me. It really hurt me – more than I admitted to my husband, Ed.

He asked me, "Are you OK?" I said yes, but my eyes had filled up with tears, which rolled down the cheeks of my face. I felt so ashamed. It was more embarrassing than anything. I felt like such a fool.

We would miss the film. I needed to change my clothes and find dressing for my wounds of my burnt hand from the hot coffee. I thought, my *God, what is wrong with me now?*

Surprise! – More Doctor Visits

Doctor Messler was an MS specialist that a neighbour in Los Angeles had recommended that I should see. I went to see this MS consultant. I had to have three more MRI scans.

Some of my old lesions were not alive or active, but there were a couple of new ones alive. This was what was causing my falls. I had to see another specialist consultant, Doctor Patel Desri, a specialist in Diet and Medication for MS patients.

He was happy with my weight and blood tests results, and also with the way I was changing my eating habits. The non-dairy and no saturated fats diet he suggested had produced results for other patients of his. It ended up that it worked quite well for me too. It is dedication to the max if you commit to fighting MS. I was giving it my all to fight back.

Good Times Along With The Rough Times

My husband and I had spoken together about us living in Los Angeles. Much of his work as a professional music producer was in LA and there were specialists I could consult with.

Yet, from the beginning, we knew America was a temporary stay for us; especially when I got seriously sick and both our families still lived in the UK.

We had got married in July of 2010 on the beautiful island of Hawaii. We stayed at the Mauna Lani Bay Resort. We were right there by the beach. We could hear the waves from the ocean hitting the rocks at the shore. It was a wonderful restful sound. It rocked my soul.

We walked together hand in hand along the white sandy beaches of South Kohala in Hawaii. It was a true paradise – clear blue sky, white sandy beaches and the deep blue of the ocean. My husband and I would go to the beach late at night just to hear the waves breaking on the sand and gaze upon the stars.

Back in Southern California we would also go to watch and hear the waves hit the shore on Hermosa Beach. Most of all, I loved to look up into the sky. Just to be in awe and wonder as the stars twinkled above, what actually the universe is made of.

We would speak softly to each other, in a state of beautiful, peaceful wonder at what is actually going on 'up there'. We shared with one another that it would be hundreds of years in the future (when we are gone) before our children's children may be able to travel to the universe above. Having holidays to the moon. Ha! Who knows?

We just rested and dreamed together on those lovely natural wonders of those beach shores. Hearing the sound of the waters, the scent of the fresh air of the sea, as the waves roll into the shore at night. I still treasure those wonderful memories.

Now, imagine a special time in *your* life. Take your thoughts there. Relax to the sound of the ocean waves crashing against the rocks at night. What was your favourite time and space from the past? What will be your most treasured time in your beautiful future? Take the time to think, dream, imagine what your life truly can be.

Your journey is far from over. Like the Winston Churchill quote at the front of the book stated, maybe this is not even the beginning. Perhaps this is just the beginning of the beginning of your renewed and healthy life. Plunge into the waters of that kind of dream.

One of my favourite quotes come from the brilliant Professor and Astrophysicist from Cambridge University (now sadly departed), Stephen Hawking. In spite of the extreme level of his disability, he always had such an open, curious mind about the makings of the universe.

Here is a jewel I often ponder when life gets overwhelming for me:

"Remember to look up at the stars, and not down at your feet. Try to make sense of what you see. And wonder about what makes the Universe exist. Be curious!!" – Stephen Hawking.

That has stuck in my mind for years. It still gives me encouragement to this day. Let's be curious about the wonderful times that await us, both in the future and in there here and now.

When It Rains It Pours – Dealing With 'Drop Foot'

I was referred to another specialist in Los Angeles that helps with issues associated with MS and Diabetes. An amazing place, called the Hanger Clinic, in Torrance, California.

The Hanger Clinic is named after James Edward Hanger. It all started with a cannonball, which James never saw coming. In the early hours of June 1861, Hanger was standing on guard in the city of Philippi, Virginia. This was the very first land battle of the American Civil War. Having been a victim of this serious injury led to poor Mr. Hanger having his leg amputated.

Now that misfortune has become a legacy for people who need help with limbs, appendages, and feet that are having problems with issues associated with them. This speciality clinic was where I went when I started experiencing 'Drop Foot' or 'Foot Drop', depending on your preference.

Drop Foot is a condition commonly associated with Multiple Sclerosis. It is a condition where the damaged nerves are unable to deliver the electrical nerve signal from our brain, when we decide we want to walk. The muscles in the ankle and foot never get the signal.

The bad thing about that is you start falling often. The body is not doing what your brain is telling it to do. It is an awful condition and can be quite dangerous.

I had a case of Drop Foot in my right foot, caused by my MS. The Hanger Clinic fitted me to have a 'Walk Aide' costing $8,000 US dollars (in 2014). It was attached to my right leg. Braced under my right knee were the electronics pads.

This Walk Aide was a pretty awesome device that assists in sending the proper electric signals to the afflicted foot. It is one of the wonderful things about where we are in combating MS, that there is research and technology being applied to helping MS sufferers cope.

The electronic pads of the Walk Aide cost $350 dollars for ten packs (at that time). This would last about ten to twelve months if used daily. The Walk Aide helps to lift your Drop Foot and helps build up the muscles again through the exercise.

It connects with my brain and the electrical impulses then help to lift my foot up as I bend my leg to walk. What that means is I can be 'stick free'. It helped me to walk independently. I will never take that for granted ever again.

Was it expensive? Yes. Was it worth it? Absolutely. Devices like this are paid out of pocket in the States. Even though it cost a lot, I was extremely thankful this technology exists.

It helped me to become more fully mobile. It helped me regain some independence. For someone who has never experienced a radical reduction to your mobility it is impossible to describe how important this is for our sense of safety and well-being.

Diabetes Can Be A Painful Death

I learned a lot from being at the Hanger Clinic in Los Angeles. Their patients had trebled over the previous couple of years. Mainly this was due to the radical increase in the number of patients with diabetes.

At its worst stages, diabetes patients are sometimes forced to have amputations of affected areas and limbs. The rate for limb amputation is very high and has doubled in the last five years. I asked my consultant in the clinic, Evan, about these things. I found out that most (not all) of diabetes is diet related.

There is has also been shown to be a connection between having Type 1 Diabetes and being three times more predisposed to acquiring Multiple Sclerosis. Though the medical research is showing some kind of connection between the two conditions, there are still many unknowns.

But this one thing we do know. Both conditions can be affected by what we choose to eat. If you would like to wait around for another two decades to see what medical research finds conclusively, then that is up to you. I would rather make some changes now. It may be wiser now to take some precautions while we still can.

Research shows definitively that diets that have high sugar levels can of course cause obesity. Obesity can make one more vulnerable to diabetes. Even little children.

With my own eyes I saw this in the clinic. It's very sad when you see young children in this clinic having artificial limbs fitted to their tiny bodies. It is very sad that problems like this are occurring at such a young age. Again, it is mainly related to eating patterns and diet.

Sugar, Carbs, and Diabetes

A change in your diet can make such significant improvements in your health. With diabetes you can do a lot with the food you eat to help reverse the conditions, or at least the symptoms of the condition.

It does take willpower and determination to heal through diet. With the significant weight loss, you can eventually come off of medications. A lot is to go with your mindset. Even if you fall, get back up again.

To combat diabetes it is recommended to go with a diet low in carbs and high in healthy, natural fats. Look at the processed foods in our stores. They contain *a lot* of carbohydrates – potatoes, rice, breads, cakes, and cereals.

Science has determined that four grams of carbs, to a diabetic, will convert to one teaspoon of sugar in your body. Having a bowl of rice will convert to 8-10 spoonsful of sugar. Only once slice of bread (it does not matter if its white or brown) will convert to four spoonsful of sugar in the body of a diabetic.

Changing (just by slightly adjusting) your choices of foods a little at a time makes such a big difference to your health. Why suffer when you do not have too?

This is important to remember; we are in charge of what goes into our mouth – unless you are in prison, you decide what passes your lips and what does not.

There is more wasted food than ever now due to the emergence of unhealthy processed foods created and distributed through the Food Industrial Complex.

Advertising trains us to 'like' these things. We over-buy them. Years ago we would grow our own crops fruit and vegetables and just picked fresh what was needed daily. No waste, and a lot healthier and cheaper.

What if every person and family had a little garden? Overweight parents and their children could work in it together to get some fun exercise, fresh air and get away from the smart phones and screens! Then they could reap the delicious fruits of their labours and pick what they want from it.

There are simple solutions to almost all of these problems. If we take the time to think about what is going on in society and ourselves, we can prevent 99% of the problems that come our way. We are resilient. We can make a change.

Gradual Change Is Lasting Change

You would not say 'no,' to being a few pounds lighter (that is, in weight not in money), right? Being a little lighter is always a nice feel-good factor. Losing some weight is one of the side benefits of eating healthy. There are many more benefits than downsides by making these changes.

Again, this natural approach is not about deprivation, or living like a monk or a nun. Make the changes gradually, but consistently. These two powerhouses of habit change work closely together.

Of course, on special occasions you can really let your hair down. You will not burst at your seams when you overindulge on a holiday like Christmas, Thanksgiving, Easter or a Halloween party. If you have some ribs at a beach barbecue, the world will not spin off its axis. Just do not eat like that every day.

Whenever you can, make recipes cooked from scratch using processed-free products. The closer to nature the better. This will prevent eating unhealthy foods without even knowing it. In these food tips and recipes, I always recommend certain kinds of foods.

To Stop or Go?

Remember though, *I am not* a Doctor, Nutritionist, or Dietician. I do not know if you have food allergies, or underlying conditions that may be contraindications for eating certain foods. You should check with your own doctor, nutritional or health consultant before making any radical dietary or medicinal changes.

To be crystal clear – I am *not* saying 'stop' if you are on a prescribed medication and it is working for you, keep on with it. I would never say something like that.

Each of our bodies is unique and individual. Perhaps for you, this natural way of life I chose to take can only help with your well-being as an extra bonus – alongside, not instead of, your prescribed medication.

Only *you* have control over what you eat. I changed my food habits. I made different choices of food and you can also. I could never imagine changing my food habits when I set out on this journey five years ago.

As I started feeling better in myself after doing so. There was less pain, fewer migraines, less wind in my stomach, and cramp pains like when I had Irritable Bowel Syndrome (IBS). It only got better when I slowly changed my old eating habits towards newer, healthier choices. I stopped craving sweets after I cut out sugar.

I could never imagine life without sugar before this diet. I used to have three heaped teaspoons of sugar in a full-fat large milk cappuccino. Now I could never go back. I now do not know how I ever took sugar, or put meat to my lips. Back then I could never imagine life without sugar or meat.

What should you stop? What new thing should you go to? This is your lesson to learn about your body. You are the only true expert on your unique individual body. I am sharing what worked for me, some basic nutritional and physiological principles. You need to really listen to that deep voice of reason within you. Learn from it. Your true body really does know what is best for you.

After you start integrating some of these dietary changes, over time your cravings will begin to change. Then you can trust it more. If you are currently craving potato crisps, beer, a chocolate bar, and a cigarette *now* – that is probably coming just from a habit. Your body really does not need any of that. Listen to what it really wants and needs. As your taste buds improve and your system cleans up a bit and gets healthier, it will let you know what it needs through real genuine cravings.

I cannot tell you how many times my tongue and tummy will crave some odd vegetable, spice, fruit or other organic food. Then when I research it, the food contains some nutritional component I actually *need*. Our natural instincts have kept humankind alive all these millennia. Maybe our bodies are not so dumb after all?

10: AROUND THE WORLD – ON A PLATE

So, come on this interesting journey around the world with me. We will be looking at the dining plates of people around the globe. *What is on their plates and how does that work out for them*?

How is it that what different peoples from around the globe put on their plates affects their disease rates and longevity? What can we learn from them as people struggling with MS and other auto-immune disorders?

You will see from these numerous countries that there is *a lot* of information that can help us in industrialized Western nations, like the UK, Europe, and the United States. We will see quite clearly what works with eating habits – *and* what does not.

Travel is always illuminating. Even more so when it comes to food. We as humans love food! It is a reflection of our nation's cultural values, a legacy of history of our innovation and survival skills, and it is embedded in our DNA. Our individual cultural heritage is also biological and physiological. Food tolerances tend to follow ethnic and cultural eating patterns.

I have studied the medical research done in many countries of the world where the people live *very* healthy and *illness-free* lives. This demonstrates to us clearly that we are what we eat.

We learn that it *is* possible to achieve a balance between work, rest, social interaction, exercise, and maintaining a balanced perspective on what is important.

We have lost that balance in most modern societies. This may be why we are sick. Time to bring that balance back. We can learn from other cultures and nations in our quest for personal development and health enhancement.

Some of these global health studies provided a numeric ranking system. It was based around research data about the nation's most common diet, average length of life, overall lifestyle and the health statistics of the peoples who live in that way.

We can learn much from studying these countries ways of life, comparing it with ours, and making the right changes where needs be. Why reinvent the wheel? Let us look at who has been doing it right and pick up some tips from them.

Top medical doctors, researchers, and dietitians from around the world will surprise you with what they have found through their research. Countries you thought would be healthy are not so, and ones you thought would be unhealthy are solid. You do not know what you do not know.

From studying fifty key countries in various global regions and their dietary patterns some commonalities were found. Let us be humble and learn from them. Our cultural way is not always the so-called 'right way' all the time.

From Africa, Asia, Latin America, Europe to the South Pacific, this is a global journey from the best and worst diets for our health. This will be like watching an Anthony Bourdain travel/eating show, only with an emphasis on the actual health outcomes of these countries' diets. And, there is no video footage. Ha! Just your rich imagination. Let us get on the rails and trails and let's get rolling on this journey.

Let us start with the Marshall Islands. This place really should be a paradise island with a *pure natural* diet. Ironically, it has the highest obesity and (surprise, surprise) growing diabetes rates globally. This is as a result mainly from cheap, fatty meats introduced into their diet recently. 70 years ago, diabetes was unheard of on this island. Now it is rampant.

Many of these developing countries have been corrupted through massive advertising campaigns to eat cheaper, imported, processed foods. They come at 'affordable prices' – yet later on in years, this comes back hard at a deadly price. The price they pay is being afflicted with chronic illnesses.

The illnesses come from the processed and imported foods. The diabetes of modern Western diets is now resulting in a high level of limb amputations in many countries. This is not coming from traditional diets based on naturally grown crops on a lovely island, but from imported processed foods.

In Russia, approximately a quarter of the men die before the age of 55. Why is that? Their preferred drink that they consume regularly in large quantities is vodka which causes liver disease and alcohol poisoning. Alcohol of course, also converts to sugar in the bloodstream. This processed, carbohydrate rich, and excessive alcohol drinking diet is killing people there.

The country of Kuwait came into wealth when they struck oil in 1938. Their society grew to *love* junk food. The same holds true for Saudi Arabia, which came in 47th in the 50 countries studies.

The 46th was the United Arab Emirates and 45th, Qatar. All of these oil rich countries in the Middle East have been negatively impacted by the influence of our modern Western diet. They are paying for it now with poor health statistics.

The traditional Middle Eastern diet is very healthy. It does not take long for nationwide dietary changes to affect the health statistics of a country. As I mentioned in my testimony, it was only one generation back that the UK was closer to nature in how we ate – from our own gardens, not a fast food 'restaurant'. Look at us now.

Mexico has a real snacking culture and there are statistics that say one in three Mexican people are obese. This is not simply due to the corn tortillas, tacos, pork, chicken, fresh salsas or other traditional Mexican foods. Unfortunately, they now have a lot of imported –and heavily-marketed – cereals, packaged foods, processed foods, and fizzy soft drinks, the same crap we have here in the UK. It has been devastating to their health.

A litre of fizzy soft drink can have up to 30 teaspoons of sugar in just one bottle. Mexicans have the highest child obesity rate in the world. Many children there are losing all their teeth far too young. The sugars go up into their 'second teeth' before they even come through.

My nephew and niece's children had too many sweets and sugary drinks growing up before they were ten years old. They had a lot of their teeth removed at once due to tooth decay. This does not just happen in developing nations. It just depends on how people eat.

Tooth Decay from Processed Foods

My children had boiled water from the time they were little babies growing up. I would give them minimal fresh fruit to snack on, or raw vegetables to eat as young children. It was easier to carry the water, rather than the juice, as I could wash their faces with it. I could even fill the car water radiator and window wash bottle! It ticked all the boxes. If they spilt it in the car, it was not sticky like juice or smelled like sour milk. Yuk!

My children are in their twenties now with not one tooth filling in their mouth, I am proud to say. I had loads of fillings in my teeth. The mercury black metal fillings done through my school dentist back in the late seventies and eighties. Thankfully, I had them removed and changed to white fillings, which is better if you have MS or other sensitive health issues.

We always had a tiny bottle of milk in our school breaks in the mornings. But there were also school '*tuck shops*,' and vending machines, sadly always full of sugary snacks and potato crisps.

You even find this mess in UK hospital's vending machines. These are all full of fizzy drinks, chocolate bars and biscuits. (all containing sugar) These types of things should be a rare treat, not everyday meals. It would be nice to see a vending machine full of fresh fruits and water someday. But that will never happen – not enough profit to be made from healthy snacks

Developing World to the Industrialized World – It Is Diet?

Good Ole USA comes in at 43rd on the list. Fast food chains kicked off strong in the USA around 1971, during the administration of President Nixon. There is a connection between food policy and health outcomes.

Tons of corn was produced, so corn syrup was added to a lot of foods. The US government spent tax dollars subsidizing the corn industry and growers, so they had to do something with all that corn to make sure their 'cash crop' came in on top economically.

Foods you would never think of often contain some high fructose corn syrup. Foods like ketchup, peanut butter, apple sauce, juices, crackers, breakfast cereal, relish and pickles; the list goes on and on.

Mass produced high fructose corn syrup (HFCS) spread around the world causing obesity. It allegedly made the foods cost less; however, it went much further than that.

This high fructose corn syrup has been heavily linked to weight gain. But, one of its most dangerous effects is how it can increase Type 2 Diabetes.

We do use far less of this in the UK than in the USA, since our food labels are required to call it what it is – high fructose corn syrup is how it shows on our ingredient's labels. So, we are more informed than our friends in the States.

The Trip Continues...

Country number 42 was Venezuela, then Argentina came in at number 41. Again, this is primarily due to imported processed foods that these countries did not score so well on overall health outcomes and longevity.

Turkey was 44th and Hungary number 39. Australia was 38th on the list. You would not expect to have a high obesity rate there. Yet, they do have it. Part of this is because of how expensive fresh vegetables and fruits are there. It is very cheap to buy processed foods in Australia and it is really, slowly killing them.

Dietary Health in The UK and British-Influenced Countries

Scotland came in at 37th and Northern Ireland 36th, where teenagers had the worst tooth decay in Europe. Mainly from the intake of sugar and fizzy soft drinks. Wales was 35th. They have a lot of the obesity among children there.

Then there is England, at 34th on the list. The rating keeps climbing higher due to the increase of obesity among young children and high rates of diabetes.

At its peak in the early 1900s, it wasn't really until the late 1950's, after wartime rationing formally ended, that the Full English or *fry-up* was regarded as the traditional breakfast. We fried bread in the bacon and sausage fat that the meats and eggs were fried in. But then, when heavily marketed breakfast cereals started to appear from the USA, we were told that the fry-up was not the best idea for one's health. In fact, compared to all the highly processed junk foods we see today, it was probably not that bad at all.

Also, at this time in the 1960's that people in the UK would have breakfast, dinner and 'tea time'. Back then only 2% of women and 1% of men were considered obese. Today, over a quarter of the population are considered medically overweight. This has to do with both reduced activity levels and of course, previously having a more naturally based diet.

There were full unintentionally 'organic' meals years ago with no snacking in between so obesity was naturally lower. The British people plucked food up from all over the world, all different kind of foods. The British people love Indian, Chinese, Japanese, and Mexican food.

Still, the English diet consists mostly of wheat, dairy, potatoes, sugars and vegetable oils. I could not believe the UK eats more ready-made-meals than any other country in Europe. I guess we are working a lot too. Probably too much.

Rapeseed oil was not really produced for food use before 'Canola Oil' (actually rapeseed) appeared in the 1970's. But, today it is now our third largest crop and this unhealthy oil is in your margarine, cooking oils and most of the processed foods out there today. It is the UK's third most common product in processed foods. Vegetables oils have taken over in a lot of our packaged foods.

'Well, it comes from plants!' Yes, it comes from plants, but when it is processed and heated, bleached, deodorised, and chemically treated, it changes the composition of many of these oils, making them really toxic for our bodies.

It used to be animal fat dripping from our meat that came from our home-cooked meals we used to eat. Today we consume more than twice as much vegetable oil than we used in the 1960's. Vegetable oils are everywhere, in so much of the processed, 'convenience' foods we now snack on, rather than our tradition of sitting down at the table with meat, two vegetables, and some boiled potatoes.

There was traditionally here in England what was called the 'Ploughman's lunch'. A simple fare of bread, cheese, a pickled onion, pickles, and a beer. If you were really rolling, you could add in the hard-boiled egg and cold sausage.

A joint of beef would have great flavour from the drippings of the fat that came from the meat. The beef of today is full of water and is tasteless from what I heard from my family.

I have not eaten meat for over six years now myself so I cannot comment on the taste of modern meat with any real authority. The UK had a lot of their own farms sold over the years. This may be affecting the quality of the meat and other food available here now.

Ranked at 33 among the 50 nations, is Ireland. They have popular beers that are lower in alcohol and calories than the beer here in the UK

The Irish drink the Irish stout beers, which is doing their health a favour in comparison to other countries. The Irish Stout beer, being lower in alcohol, is healthier. Their most famous Irish stout, Guinness, claims it is also high in iron.

The Rest of The World's Countries Ratings

Uruguay came in rated at number 32. This is a country where a quarter of their adult population are overweight. The story here started in 1840, when German scientist, Justus von Liebig, came up with the idea condensing three kilos of meat into just 100 grams of powder.

He was the person who gave birth to the mighty 'stock cube'. He set his factory up in Uruguay. He chose a small town called, 'Fray Bentos' and one of the most popular UK ready-meals was born: 'Fray Bentos – a pie in a tin.'

I remember having seen this growing up. They used to be kept in the larder cupboard at 'Nan's' house. It was a pie in a tin. A form of condensed corned beef. My nan would cut the round tin open. There was a whitish pastry. It never looked very good to me!

This thing would come out of the oven, golden brown like a puff pastry top in a tin swimming in thick beef gravy. These easy-to-prepare 'ready meals' were a long way from a fresh, home cooked meal that most English working class people were used to getting.

Now, there are all sorts of ways that people in the UK end up eating these unnatural meat concoctions. Too many of our luncheon meats, canned meats, packaged meats are being used a lot for convenience, but are not healthy for us at all.

Processed Meats Are Not Good For You

There are processed meats we buy to make sandwiches. So many different meats that have been processed and treated with preservatives. Meats like bacon, ham, sausages, pressed chicken, smoked turkey, salami, etc. The list is endless. For your health it is best to limit these as much as you can.

Instead, consider using meat leftovers from a cooked roast to make sandwiches. Even canned tuna, sardines, or pilchards would be better than processed luncheon meats.

You can always have hard-boiled eggs, mixed with salt, pepper, and chopped fresh cherry tomatoes. You can have chicken leftover from a roast, mixed with avocado, salt, and black cracked pepper. But probably best to skip the mayonnaise as that is usually made from up to 80% rapeseed oil!

Limit the amount of red meat in your diet. If you do eat red meat, try doing so only once or twice a week. Better yet, switch it out for a 400g round of lamb or goat curry. Try that to replace the pork and beef. By doing this, you will reduce your risk of a lot of cancers. There has been evidence that processed meats and too much red meat has been linked to a bowel cancer and liver cancer.

You do need a certain amount of protein in your daily diet. We need it to keep our bodies well and to repair our cells. Eat half a plate of green vegetables, then add other items like healthy organic rice or potatoes pasta. We can replace the proteins of meat with those of legumes, grains, etc.

What have you learned so far from taking this global trip around the world on a plate? We have learned that a lot of what modern industrialized countries are eating is potentially deadly to them, and the countries they import this food off to are suffering as well.

What are some better ways to eat and live? Let us explore some solutions as we get back on the bus in the next chapter. We have new worlds of health and taste to explore!

11: WHAT IS THE BEST WAY TO LIVE?

What Are The Secrets to A Long Healthy Life?

Now our trip is moving towards the *best* foods and diets in the world and to the secrets for a long healthy life. Sit back in your chair as we continue this tour of world via their plates – what are other everyday people around the globe eating? And how is it affecting their health and longevity?

North Africa

Ethiopia is the 24th healthiest country in this research. This is a country with a lush array of natural fresh from the farm foods. Ethiopia is still an agricultural based society. They grow a lot there, from chilli peppers to legumes, dried beans and clean grains.

Historically, Ethiopia has grown this one major grain. The name of this wonder seed is called '*Teff*'. Teff is made up a tiny grain of a seed so fine it looks like a grain of sand.

This grain with the tiny seeds has a lot of iron, fibre, and protein in it. It is actually made up of two-thirds protein. '*Injera*', the pancake-like bread made from the teff grain with a delicious sourdough-like flavour is the Ethiopian peoples' staff of life.

Injera is used like a gentle wrap, where seasoned lentils, greens, vegetables, and legumes and placed in and eaten with the hands. Occasionally there will be some fish, chicken, or beef, but percentage wise, they do not really eat much meat. Their diet is mostly healthy, protein-rich grains and vegetables, so they have a low risk of colon cancer.

Morocco was rated number at 20. This is a country which has the lowest recorded rates of liver cancer in the world. They do not do drink alcohol as their religion (Islam) forbids it. Instead, they drink lots of fresh mint tea. Naturally, this would make sense.

East Asia

China is rated 18th on the list of healthy countries. China is the most populated country in the world. This is a bit of a surprise, since white rice on its own is not that healthy. It causes a spike your blood sugar levels in your body. But the Chinese combine their rice with a lot of different fresh vegetables. This then releases the sugar more slowly into the system. Chinese people consume 40 percent more vegetables than we eat here in the UK or USA. *This* is why their diet came in so high in healthiness, not the white rice they eat.

Indonesia is number 17 on the list and Malaysia is 16th. Number 15 is Vietnam. These four countries (including China) share rice as their grain staple. But rice, *along with* numerous fresh vegetables mixed with fresh herbs, and hot chilli peppers, speed up your metabolism and release endorphins – the pleasure hormone. Preparation makes a big difference in the healthy quality of foods that we eat.

South Korea is 13th on the list, and counting down. This country is doing it right with their diet. South Korea has one of the lowest obesity rates in the world. Their people stay slim. Part of it is the raw fish they eat a lot. They also eat fresh octopus and many other kinds of fresh seafood.

They have fresh produce in their vegetable stands and they eat virtually no dairy. People there are about 90 percent lactose intolerant in Korea. This is a common digestive problem where your body is unable to digest lactose, a type of sugar mainly found in milk and dairy products. The nasty effects normally start about 2-3 hours after ingesting the diary.

In South Korea vegetables are king. They actually consume double the amount of vegetables per person than we eat in the UK. Korea's biggest national dish is '*Kimchi*', eaten at almost every meal. Kimchi is a fermented cabbage. Although it's high in sodium (like pickles) kimchi contains very healthy bacteria for your digestion – probiotics.

The longer the kimchi ferments, the higher the amount of Vitamin B-12. Koreans have been eating kimchi for centuries. South Korean people actually work the longest hours in the world. They are on their smartphones 24/7. Yet, these people really do stay close to their original tradition of food and life style.

Their life style is super busy, very hectic, so you have no excuse to make up! Just try to do what they do. Eat some really good healthy foods. Make dishes from fresh ingredients. Eat mostly lots and lots of vegetables. It is pretty simple really.

Sri Lanka is number 12 in the world of healthy diets. Their secret? Sri Lanka is a lovely island where they use a massive amount of coconut milk in a lot of their foods. This lowers the bad cholesterol and increases good cholesterol.

India is number 11 in the world. It actually used to be one colonies of the United Kingdom. In our 'take away foods' we British people really love a good Indian dish. It is one of the most popular restaurants for people in the UK to go to. Their key to health may be turmeric. This root is an ingredient which has been shown to be very anti-inflammatory and can even possibly prevent cancer.

The Diverse Diets of Europe

Spain is ninth on the countries and Spanish ladies are the second longest living ladies, right after Japanese women. Is it the red wine in the diet? The freshness of their food? The 'siestas'?

France is really is an impressive country. The French are at number eight of fifty countries with the healthiest diets. The French people in Toulouse have a better heart rate than the UK, even though they eat loads of cheese, meat, and wine. Why is that?

Nutritionists and medical researchers call this paradox of high fat (and healthy) diet creating a healthy population in France, the 'French Paradox.' The French generally have low levels of cholesterol. Is it the red wine?

Research from Cambridge suggest that the mold on the Blue Cheese is like a 'Rock Ball' rolling though our system. The mold seems to act as an anti-inflammatory within the system in our bodies. The French have up to three thousand different cheeses! French people eat cheese every day. Yet, the French are so healthy.

The French have low levels of heart disease. They have three meals a day – average to smaller size meals, with no snacking. They may take one or two hours to sit and eat these meals slowly, sitting down with friends, enjoying the foods over a glass or two of red wine. They enjoy their foods and take their time.

Some researchers speculate that it is perhaps *how they eat*, rather than *what they eat* that may be the reason behind the French Paradox. Taking time to eat slowly is a big boost to healthy digestion, which means healthy elimination, which means less toxins in our bodies.

Many Britons regularly consume pre-packaged sandwiches, potato crisps, snack bars and fizzy drinks that get lumped into the 'Meal Deal.' Rather than taking our time eating, we (like the Americans) grab 'fast food'. Even the French say eating this way is dangerous.

Nordic Countries, like Sweden, Norway, and Denmark are unique. Danish chefs have been taking the world by storm. Their traditional diet is rich in oats and rye, berries, raspberries, blueberries, salmon and seasonal vegetables. It is sometimes called the 'Mediterranean Diet' of the North. All healthy good stuff – and lots of '*Superfoods.*'

Japanese Traditional Diet

Japan has a diet bursting with health benefits from all their fresh fish and lots of vegetables. The Japanese come in fifth in this list. But their beloved soy sauce is high in sodium and is linked to strokes, which is a common cause of death in Japan. Yet Japan's cuisine is big on vegetables, fruit and fish and their longevity is quite high.

The Healthy Mediterranean Diet

Greece and Italy were number three and two on the list of global healthy diets. These diets roughly fall into the category of the famous 'Mediterranean diet.'

The lifestyle in Campodimele in Italy is studied by longevity experts. People live longer there, since they are physically active all day long. They cultivate their own food, working in the fields by tending olive groves, herding sheep and goats and growing grapes and wine.

They engage in *lots* of walking or cycling up and down their steep hillsides. They are exposed to plenty of sunshine – this keeps their anti-cancer vitamin D levels up. The air is fresh there too. The environment can play a big role.

They go to bed at dusk and rise at dawn. This helps keep their hormones young with a good eight-plus hours sleep a night. Going to bed at the same time every night improves our circadian rhythms and especially adrenal function if you suffer from insomnia. This will have profound effects on your physical and mental health.

We need to get as much fresh air as possible. We all need to get out on a regular basis to the countryside, to breathe sea air, or fresh mountain air. Many Italians also normally take a 'siesta' after lunch. Campodimele is nicknamed the place of 'Long Genetics,' since their *average* life expectancy is 95 years.

In Italy, many people even make their own olive oil. Apart from lowering your bad cholesterol it can lower your risks getting of Alzheimer's disease. A combination of an overall low consumption of red meat, lots of olive oil, and eating fresh vegetables lowers your blood pressure.

Of their delicious red wine, the Italians drink two glasses every day, but nothing in the evening. They make their own pasta from scratch. There is much we can learn from this lovely country with some of the most delicious cuisine in the world. The Italians simple lifestyle, simple fresh foods, and slower pace bears lessons for all of us, regardless of where we happen to be on the planet.

And Number 1... Iceland – Seriously?

Iceland, remarkably is the number one country in the world on diet and health. Men live the longest there, to an average of age 81. Icelanders eat plenty of wild fish; salmon, halibut and even shark, all rich in Omega 3's. Fish can also help with depression. Not eating enough fish has been linked to mental health issues such as Alzheimer's and Schizophrenia.

Iceland is an isolated country. They also there is lack of pollution due to their unique geothermal activity, relative isolation, and lower population. Pollution can have profoundly harmful poisonous effects on populations. The level of pollution in the air is rising here in UK. Are we trying to catch up to Los Angeles?

Apparently, the natural geothermal heat from the volcanic landscape helps reduce the pollution levels in Iceland. Going to the hot tubs makes you healthy. People like to go from the hot water, to laying on the ice and putting snow on their bodies. Then they jump back into the hot tub and back into the elements. All this is healthy for the muscles all the way down into the nerves of the body. It can also reduce inflammation.

Many Icelanders take cod liver oil every day, around a teaspoon and they eat a lot of rye bread. Clean healthy grains are a big part of a healthy diet. Wholegrain bread and pasta is better for diabetics. Though the dietary patterns of Iceland may be strange, they seem to have the best diet in the world for your health.

Icelanders eat fish like crazy. If you eat fish raw you get a 10 out of 10 nutritionally. The original raw state of fish both looks and tastes fantastic. Fish, if you steam it, the vitamins left are about an 8 out of 10 nutritionally. If you fry it in a pan you lose even more vitamins. About a 6 out of 10. Deep fried fish is left with less than half of its vitamins, at about a 4 out of 10 nutritional points.

If you do decide to eat red meats, use high quality meats, ethically treated, and raised on natural non-GMO feed and grasses. Grass-fed cow's milk is best for your hair, eyes and skin. Lambs being grass fed, are less fatty and full of Omega 3's. Yes, it is more expensive, but how expensive will it be to treat your sick body?

What Have We Learned From The World's Plates?

So here we are back at home. What have we learned? What are we to make of all of this? The French eat loads of cheese, which is high in saturated fat. Ethiopians eat hardly any meat at all – almost exclusively grains like teff, lentils, and vegetables.

The Koreans eat loads of vegetables. The Mediterranean Diet communities indulge in olive oil. Lots of cultural, geological, and environmental differences. What are the commonalities that lead to longevity, health, and a better quality of life?

They all have this one thing in common: Very few processed foods.

They follow traditional dietary eating patterns with mostly fresh from the farm diets. They have a dedication of eating a minimal amount of over processed, non-traditional foods. They basically eat and live as their ancestors did for hundreds, and some, thousands of years. They seem to follow the model in their lifestyle and diet, 'If it ain't broke, don't fix it.'

I have taken this approach to diet and eating to a new level. A new lifestyle that is really an 'old' lifestyle. To your beating heart it does not matter where you live in the world. It is *how you live* that matters. We can all be eating the world's 'best diet' *anywhere* in the world these days, if you just follow these core principals of choosing your food.

These countries healthy statistics and delicious cuisines have proven that there is life without processed foods. The food industry's advertising hype and colourful packaging seeks to influence you to buy their manufactured junk. Not junk *food*. It is barely that; it is just junk... *food-like substances*. The onslaught of their propaganda is everywhere from TV commercials, to posters on buses and subways, the underground and tube stations, and on the internet. Big money is made out of cheap foods. Big advertising dollars too.

Take away the cakes, sweets, crackers, especially those full of sugar, and potato crisps, all of which are full of unhealthy fats. Skip the drinks high in sugar. If you do consume these they should be in small amounts only, like alcohol.

So, great mysteries solved!

The key to a long life is a *simple life*; staying really fit and eating naturally and healthily. Simply put, a healthy life is to live off of the land. All fresh vegetables, rich in legumes, whole grains, fruit, fish and limited red meats.

So how feasible is it for you to do that from where you are from? You may not be able to follow such a lifestyle as perfectly as people can in some of these regions. But you can improve. You can drop some old eating and lifestyle habits that no longer serve you (or your condition). Then, you can start some new habits that will help you. It is as simple as that.

12: GETTING BACK IN BALANCE

Sugar and fat are the key problems with the Western diet. How do we repair the damage once it is done? You can start to repair your nerves and your damaged cells though what you eat. Like I have done over the last few years. Good 'brain food' will produce new cells in your brain and nervous system.

By taking fish oil capsules regularly, research has shown a decrease in MS relapse rates. I freeze my capsules, and swallow them frozen. It can also help reduce the repeating of fish meals too often if the costs of buying fish regularly is a factor.

Having MS means we have more fatty acids. There has been research and a range of evidence regarding polyunsaturated fatty acids. Omega-3 and Omega-6 are Fatty Acids and these two may have therapeutic effects for MS patients. We need to eat more of them and less saturated fats.

Cutting out saturated fats has been shown to decrease and reduce production of inflammation. Research studies are showing clinical improvement in the levels of inflammation by eliminating these from our diets.

The food I have eaten over the last five years has helped me repair some of my brain cells. I continue to keep up to date with setting MRI tests and I follow through with my regular medical check-ups.

Managing the monster of MS successfully comes from setting small goals and following through on those steps. One step at a time, soldier. The same way we got here is the same way we get out; one step at a time. Do not be overwhelmed. We will break this down into bite-sized chunks.

Good Brain Food Helps Our Whole System

We have to eat a lot of 'brain berries'. These contain Polyphenols. Polyphenols are so good for your body. Incredibly powerful energy boosters. They are loaded inside dark berries. They are powerful at fighting inflammation, reducing joint pain and they boost your metabolism. It keeps you younger, too!

Polyphenol is a natural plant food source that has antioxidants.

As a group they help to protect the cells in your body from free radical damage. The main thing is that these antioxidants can reduce inflammation and slow the growth of tumours. In plants, polyphenol help defends against attacks by insects and they give plants their colour. They will help protect you too.

Polyphenols have been studied by scientists. They balance your cholesterol and reduce wind and bloating. Intestinal gas will occur as a natural by-product from food digestion.

Bloating occurs when your stomach swells up from the gas. It feels like it has been enlarged when your stomach feels very full. These undigested foods allow more bacteria into in your colon. Drinking plenty of water is very good for flushing out your system and can help with gas and bloating.

Blackberries have beneficial effects on your brain health and digestive system. Blackberries can really fill you up and blackberries and blueberries support heart health. They also contain potassium, vitamin C and fibre. Having fibre content is critical.

Blueberries help reduce the amount of cholesterol in your blood and decreases the risk of heart attacks and cancer. Blueberries are also anti-inflammatory.

Blueberries also help protect the brain from oxidative stress and may also reduce the effects of age-related conditions such as Alzheimer's disease or dementia. Remember, blueberries cooked in baked oats or pancakes will not have as much nutritional value as ones eaten raw.

Strawberries are high in vitamin C. Eight strawberries will provide you with more vitamin C than an orange. This fruit has the antioxidants and they are also a good source of manganese and potassium. These trace minerals have numerous health benefits for our blood sugar and bone health.

Raspberries are an excellent of vitamin C, magnesium, and dietary fibre. They are also a good source of vitamin K. There are a load of antioxidants and phytonutrients in these berries.

Mulberries are also rich in vitamin C. They can increase your immunity to fight against common diseases, such as colds, flu or many similar infections. Mulberry can also improve vision. This fruit is an all-round strengthener and nourishes hair growth and are used to prevent early greying of your hair. Mulberries are the best tonic to increase memory and promotes a healthy brain. Being very rich in fibre they can improve digestion, and thus prevent constipation. Some suggest that mulberries provide you with health benefits to protect from some forms of cancer.

These healthy 'brain berries' will prevent a sharp rise and sugar levels this will help you if you have diabetes. It also strengthens the nervous system to become stronger and reduces bad cholesterol, thus it prevents blockage in the flow of your blood. Good fruits prevent heart attacks and strokes. If you are smart, you will eat them on the regular.

Powerful Superfood Seeds

I consume about 40 grams of chia whole seeds per day. These tiny black and white seeds are a big energy booster. These seeds are a concentrated food containing a healthy mixture of Omega -3 acids, complex carbohydrates, proteins, fibre, antioxidants, and calcium. You can mix them into your yoghurt.

I like them mixed with 40 grams of organic jumbo oats and a tablespoon of chia seed. Cover with water in a cereal bowl in the microwave for just 2 minutes. Then leave to stand to cool a minute or so. You can add banana or blueberries and strawberries on the top. Delicious!

Very filling and very good for your brain also. Chia seeds are a natural source of folic acid. They are gluten-free and vegan source of protein, all with iron, zinc, and high in good polyunsaturated fats. They are great in a smoothie!

Just one portion of chia seeds daily contains enough Omega-3 ALA to help maintain healthy cholesterol levels. It has worked for me, ever since I have been adding to my daily food intake. My blood tests have shown a big improvement in my cholesterol levels.

What Could You Use To Feel 'Super Charged?'

After you eat berries or Chia seeds you will feel 'super-charged'. They can help counter heart disease. Studies in the last 12 years show that polyphenols help you get good health in your heart.

There are other fruits loaded with polyphenols.

Apples, apple juice, pomegranates, peaches, blood orange juice, lemon juice, apricots, quince. Superfoods make each mouthful count. Make them a key part of your diet.

Eat unlimited vegetables, unlimited fruits, and plenty of summer fruits, which are delicious! Eat lots of white fish, and organic grains like rye, barley, and wheat.

Eat lots of legumes, like beans and lentils. They have great fibre and protein. Eat lots of the pea family legumes. Eat lots of seeds like flaxseed, celery seeds, etc. In the nut family you have chestnuts, hazelnuts, pecans, almonds, and walnuts. What a feast that nature has provided us!

Then in the wonderful olive family you have the most benefits – you have black olives, green olives and olive oil. All good, just be mindful of the sodium levels in pre-packaged olives.

Good vegetables are globe artichokes, red chicory, green chicory, red onion, spinach, broccoli and curly endive. These will all give your system a kick – for the good. We could all use an energy boost.

By choosing these kinds of healthy organic vegetables and super-foods, we can bypass so many of the digestive ailments that afflict people in the western industrialized societies. Ask yourself, is the pain really worth it?

Digestive Problems

Think about when you feed a cat or dog. They go to the toilet not long after they had eaten. Humans somehow think it's OK to go just once a day to the big toilet. It is not OK really. Try detoxing your body and you will see the health difference.

Notice how a baby always goes to a 'number 2' toilet after they have been fed. That is natural. When you are young you have more hydrochloric acid in our digestive system. Hydrochloric acid tends to decline as we get older.

To not be 'regular' in our elimination leads to poor health. This is what helps to create toxins to build up in our system. This problem will occur when the stomach is unable to produce enough hydro-chloric acid to meets the body's digestive needs.

This will happen more often beginning in your 40's, as the acid starts to decline more. Fatty foods, meats, and other hard to digest products causes this fermenting, making the digestive process more of a strain.

Then people can develop 'acid reflux' and they then have to take Gaviscon, or other over-the-counter stomach antacids. Then there is the constant coughing when your body attempts to keep releasing gas. It is OK to belch, before and after a meal but, you are not getting rid of the problem. You are just putting a temporary lid on it.

Meat Putrefies in Your Stomach – Meat Substitutes

Meat can apparently take up to 3 to 4 hours to digest, then another 4-6 hours to leave your body through your elimination. This means that meat sits in your gut for a *very* long time. If you stop eating meat, then you will need to take vitamin B12 supplements.

It has been proven scientifically that when you have cancer, it may be helpful to cut out or, radically cut down your intake of meat. If you have cancer you are often even told to cut out the dairy. Moving to a plant-based diet can be helpful when combating cancer.

At the end of the day, slowly reduce down these things, 'like for like'. Change it out for anything plant based that make things taste like meat. By replacing, 'like for like' you do not feel as if you are depriving yourself, or missing out on anything.

You can change a meat burger for a veggie or portobello mushroom burger. The same with other meat-like replacements such as tofu, seitan, etc. There are many plant based foods that can replace the taste of meat.

Oesophagus Health – Acid Reflux

My husband would have this at times. He would eat fried fatty foods, causing the stomach acid to back up into his oesophagus bringing back up some of the acid from his stomach. This can be terribly painful. It got to the point with my husband that he burst his oesophagus.

Then he would have to drink *Gaviscon*, or take similar antacid tablets. Rather than go through all of that, try to control yourself and eat more healthily. Conditions like this deplete your whole immune system. But taking antacids or other drugs that only address the particular issue is merely putting a temporary lid on the problem.

Colon Polyps and Cancer

Colon and rectal cancer are a major health problem in the USA. They are actually the second biggest killer of men. Yet, it is treatable if caught in time. A colon polyp can often enlarge if there is a lack of fibre to clean them out. This may develop into other forms of cancer.

It is absolutely worth having check-ups! Your first colonoscopy should be around your 'nifty-fifty' birthday. If a direct family member has had cancer, then it's recommended you have a check in the 'naughty-forties.' Bottom line? Eat right and get the check-ups.

What to Avoid Eating – Prevention Is Better Than Cure

Try to Never Eat:

Processed meat products, egg yolks, commercial cakes, definitely most fast food/takeaway meals and dairy products. Lectins can potentially cause leaky gut, to joint pains which makes this to be worse than gluten. Skip margarine and 'spreads', and foods fried in bad oils such as vegetable oils.

A lot of the 'never eat' list are processed 'white colour' foods – dairy, milk, butter, yoghurt, eggs, white bread, commercial biscuits, white flour products, and refined sugar.

I stopped eating saturated fats. I do not buy them now. I would not say my shopping bill is cheaper, but it is healthier. Having MS, you do need to stay off saturated fats. This includes animal fat products such as cream, cheese, butter, other whole milk dairy products, and fatty meats. They all contain dietary cholesterol.

There are certain vegetable products which have high saturated fat content, such as coconut oil and palm kernel oil. Consume these in moderation (though, coconut oil is great for skin health).

Never eat chocolate (as much as we love it) in sweets and ice cream. Crisps/potato chips are out, chocolate drinks, and sugary sweets. Strongly caffeinated, and/or high sugar beverages such as sweetened coffee, tea and soft drinks are also a no-no.

If you suffer from acne try keeping off of the dairy and milk products. Just begin by knowing about your foods. Milk has a lot of problems. It can cause the body to produce a lot of insulin when you consume dairy milk. Many cultures tend to be lactose-intolerant. If you love milk, what can you replace it with?

You can also choose rice milk, coconut milk, and almond milk. These can replace the dairy milks and products. Your taste buds always have to get used to new things and their different tastes so introduce them gradually.

Other foods to avoid are any potato crisps. Apart from these crisps being fried in nasty, unhealthy oils, crisps and white potatoes contain too many bad carbs. This can also can lead to an insulin spike. Crisps are one of the worst products on the market that ruin your skin and damage your health. These are a big cause of skin problems, such as acne.

Bread can also be problematic. Gluten in bread increases inflammation which is one of the main triggers of acne in many people. It is called Coeliac Disease and if you are allergic to gluten it can have severe reactions in the digestive system and the skin. You can get a medical test to see if you have it, since it is considered to possibly be genetic.

Chocolate, as delicious as it is, can cause problems with the skin. The main problem with it is the sugar. The sugar rush will play havoc with your skin. The darker the chocolate, the lower the sugar and dairy. It is also critical to avoid fizzy drinks, ice cream, and other high sucrose foods if you want to improve the health of your body, skin, and overall system.

I really try my best not to eat processed foods. Now with MS, it plays havoc with my stomach and I feel very tired, fatigued, with 'no energy syndrome' a little while after I have eaten food that is not within my regular plan. It is simply not worth it.

Try cutting out sugar and do not use a substitute. I made that mistake before. Now, after five years, if sugar is added to my drinks it tastes yucky! It makes me shiver. I always had a sweet tooth, which is the reason why I used to love coffee over tea (with tea, I never took sugar in it at first.) Now and again I will have coffee – just black; no sugar and no milk.

How Can You Make So Many Changes?

First of all, cut down *slowly*. Do not beat yourself up over anything. But you will notice the difference and will not believe at all, that you ever took sugar or milk in your tea or coffee.

It is funny really, because if you were blindfolded and served certain foods or drinks, you could not tell the difference. Unless you saw them with your eyes, then you would really enjoy them.

A lot of our feelings in food taste do start with our eyes. Sight, mind, then taste. Some foods do not look tasty since they are not decorated in bright, sugary, coloured sweetness to make our mouth water in temptation.

Over the last five years I cut one item out of my food plan at a time, say, every three months. That would be only four big changes in one year. No big deal! So over five years, I have cut out twenty items I used to have on a regular basis. We are creatures of habit, we humans. Make change easy and do not push it too hard. Then the change may last a lifetime.

So, What Can We Eat?

The Power of Vegetables

Over half of your plate should be vegetables. They have the bulk of the vitamins your body needs. I consume over half my plate daily of fresh vegetables. And, most of the time, organic vegetables.

Try cooking them lightly steamed so they retain more of the vitamins. The less you cook the vegetables, the better. Imagine it with marks out of ten – Crunchy are an 8, slightly crunchy a 5, soft vegetables a 3, and mashed vegetables a 0. We want the higher score.

Not all the goodness of healthy organic vegetables will stick around. It depends on how they are cooked, since all the vitamins may go off into the water or oil. The reason you buy good organic vegetables are the more plentiful vitamins. They have essential nutrients in limited amounts. Cook them carefully.

The greener the vegetable, generally the better the content of vitamins. Cooking vegetables lightly has helped my MS symptoms. While I wait for the vegetables to steam I leave a few raw vegetables – like carrots, sugar snap peas etc., just to snack on. It was so easy to snack on biscuits! Now I snack mostly on veggies.

Just remember to eat at a lot of green vegetables – the greener the better. As I shared above, do not overcook your green vegetables. Retain the greenish water from the greens to make a healthy soup stock (you can store it in your freezer). It can be the best part of the soup!

It is critical in protecting our cardiovascular system to regulate our blood sugar levels. We do this by eating a lot of vegetables, fruits, healthy proteins and complex, protein rich grains. So what should be some of the core items in our daily diets? Focus on ramping up the number and variety of vegetables you consume each day.

You need five portions of fruit or vegetables at a minimum daily. Choose unsaturated fats and oils if you are cooking them. These provide fibre which is essential and keeps your digestive system moving. Fibre is in so abundant in plant-based foods, just like whole meal bread, fruit, vegetables, and many pulses.

Where Are The Snacks?

Need something sweet? Have a sorbet, instead of a diary ice cream. Medjool dates are delicious sweets for snacking! They are rather nutritious and, rumour has it, good for the reproductive system.

I love pumpkin seeds for potassium and vitamin E. For a chocolate drink, I take cocoa. For biscuits/crackers, I use fat free ones. I choose whole meal, gluten-free, wheat-free bread, or sourdough bread. I love Italian Ciabatta bread, which uses olive oil.

For my cereals I make my own muesli: organic oats, a few mixed nuts, and sunflower seeds high in vitamin E and thiamine. This is high in phosphorus. Low phosphorus levels will manifest as bone issues, pain, muscle weakness, and fatigue in your body.

If you like Kale (which I love) try this recipe for 'Kale Crisps':

On a baking tray place some chopped kale. Sprinkle it with little extra virgin olive oil and a little hot chilli powder. Bake in oven until crisp. Gas 6, electric oven 180c. (350 degrees Fahrenheit.) These are the kale crisps to snack on. Yummy!

My favourite Smoothie is this:

Some Almond milk, a quarter cup of Chia Seeds, and a little golden syrup. Put this into the fridge overnight. Then blend in the morning. It is quick, simple and delicious!

I love my Tea! I use herbal teas. Instead of potato crisps I eat nuts and some dried fruit, or vegetables chopped into sticks. Use Honey instead of sugar, good quality honey.

I most definitely try to avoid those things that I know are going to make me feel lethargic or sluggish. I have the power to choose what to eat. Now, I choose to fill my plate with 'feel good' nutritious foods. This is an easy and wise way to fire up on all cylinders and give your starved body some nutrition.

I have chosen different kinds of recipes to help non-dairy and dairy eaters. For us MS people, it is important to take away the dairy and saturated fats from our bodies. This alone has been helping my cells heal themselves.

You need protein in your food choices to repair your cells. It helps in making new cells grow where they have been damaged, or have died, through any neurological conditions. With MS I eat a lot of fish. It is in my top choice of foods.

If you are a meat eater you can eat fish or chicken. Consume very little red meat. When I cook with meat (which is rare, mostly for guests) I curry goat, or lamb. It has to be the very best cut of meat. Honestly, I now prefer Tofu or other meat substitutes.

It is worth it to buy organic. I choose to have smaller food portions, but of higher quality. I eat *good* food, not *a lot* of food. Processed meats will never again be on my menu.

I do not want MS to define me. I just want to live *harmoniously* with MS, we do have to live together. I need to work with its rhythms. It is about respecting your one precious body. Your body should be your temple – if you want it to last. Some days I forget I have MS. On other days I feel fatigue, tiredness, and numbness also. It then reminds me to *listen* to my body.

Change is very possible. If you believe you can, you are halfway there. Motivation, willpower, and dedication. You can make these changes! You can heal yourself. It is like learning to walk again, slowly to build your body and making your weak muscles strong again.

Any illness makes us weak and tired. I can say I have been around family and friends with the flu, or some kind of cough or sore throat infections. I can honestly say that by eating well, buying natural fresh foods that are corn syrup free, lactose free, gluten free and dairy free products I have been infection-free for the last five years!

Before I was constantly tired, bloated and just felt unwell. I am not a doctor, but I know by my own experiences in the past, it has not all been put down due to the MS. Still, with no stomach problems from bacteria, no urine infections, or cystitis. That is good!

The long and short is, MS is becoming very common in the Western world, along with many other neurological illnesses. These are all on the increase even among own children. And it will be in our children's children. There is no cure for MS but, you can prevent such an illness – beginning in the first place with your diet and lifestyle.

Start by detoxing on your own, steadily and slowly. Just be mindful and careful. Listen to what your body is telling you. You may want to keep a food diary and write down everything that passes through your mouth into your system.

Do this for a week, or maybe even over a month. In doing so, you will surprise even yourself about what you feed your machine. By integrating these changes one at a time, you will be counteracting the degeneration of our illness. You will get stronger. And speaking of getting stronger, it is time to get physical (Can you hear Olivia Newton-John's song, 'Let's Get Physical'?). Good. *Let's Get Physical.*

13: LET'S GET PHYSICAL

Time to Look After Yourself

Strive to get yourself active in physical exercise. By getting physical you make yourself flexible so bending becomes easy again, without strain or breaking a bone. Getting physical will loosen tight, stiff muscles. This one thing – regularly getting physically active has profoundly helped me cope with my MS symptoms.

The exercise classes I choose to go to regularly are Pilates, Hydro Power, MS Chair Fit, swimming, and oxygen therapy. All these exercises together done each week have given me stability, energy, and balance *without* using sticks over the last two years. I can assure you, my readers, to me, this is nothing short of a miracle.

We always make excuses not to exercise and that it is not the right time. "I'll start next week, next month" etc., which of course, never comes. Regular exercise will be worth your while. I am not ever giving up on exercise and physical activity... Not ever.

You say you do not have money for a gym membership. First of all, you do not need one. You can move for free in your house, by doing Tai Chi, Qigong, yoga, or callisthenics. But if you think you do need a gym, seriously think about how much cash you have wasted over the years on items you no longer have.

For example, think of the depreciation of a brand-new car you may have bought. When it is driven out of a show room, all that money you lost. Think of furniture you no longer have that you have had to throw out, or have given away. Consider investing that kind of money into exercise classes – where the results are lasting.

Exercise is an important factor in creating our own good health. We have to keep our bodies moving. I love to workout in an exercise class; its sociable, the time flies past, it is never boring (far from it). It is so much fun.

Just being more active is the way to go. Try taking the stairs instead of an escalator or lift. I am experiencing a wonderful penthouse with amazing views. When I can I take the stairs. I really look forward to the stairs. It has helped strengthen my legs and actually toned them.

I would rather take the stairs than a lift or escalator.

Hydro Power Exercise Class

I love going to Hydro Power class on a Monday morning at Cascades Leisure Centre in Gravesend. I leave home at 8am and take to the road as I have a bit of a drive to get there. It is worth every moment to get into the pool and start those activities. We exercise to music and I do love Hydro Power in the water. You do not have to be a swimmer to attend as there is the shallow end of the pool. We exercise to moving 80's music.

It is about a 45-minute workout and the groups are awesome! Very helpful if I had a bad day – that wonderful social support. I have been going for a couple of years now. Victoria Bruce, our instructor, has got the class so large that it is now often booked far in advance.

I also attend on a Wednesday class for 45 minutes and sometimes Friday classes too. When I first started it was very difficult for me. My friend, Bettie Carole, would some days help me into and out of the water after the exercise.

Carole has an aunt who she has seen over the years. This aunt has had her struggles with MS too so Carole understands the pattern; there can be some bad days. Nothing can be taken for granted, especially life itself.

'Chair-Fit' Exercise Class

Lots of lovely stretching using different parts of your body and muscles. On a Monday it is a full-on two and a half hours of exercise! It is really worth trying one of these classes if they are available in your region.

Pilates

Emma Staples is an excellent Pilates instructor. She plays soft music in the background, soothing you as you exercise. The classes have been going for over 20 years at the Swanscombe Leisure Sports Centre. in an area where I used to live and so have been training in a Saturday morning class. A sharp start at 9am in the morning. It has always been so much fun with her – respect to a wonderful trainer.

Emma seeks achievement for us all; she really cares about her group. People are often advised to take up Pilates to strengthen their core which is great for balance, especially when struggling with MS.

Pilates realigns your body. Why wait until you get an injury before you go? Since I have been going I have really learned to understand my body and how much we stoop over. It is really something to sit up straight – shoulders back. Unfortunately, we often hunch our shoulders around when sitting on a sofa. That may feel comfortable for the moment, but it can also throw our spine alignment out.

Ivan Beadle is another Pilates Instructor on Wednesday mornings at Cascades Leisure Centre – he has over 20 years of experience. There are 36 different movements in Pilates.

They even teach line dancing; another way of keeping fit! Or why not try a karate or other martial arts class?

The 'A to Z's' of Getting Fit

You still remember your ABCs, right? So this should be an easy and simple way to break out of the box with the many ways we can get healthy activity and exercise. Ponder this and then pick one or two to experiment with. This is all about you re-learning to have fun moving.

A = ACTIVE: Do your housework or climb a set of stairs.

B = BORING is your enemy. Do something which is really fun for you.

C = CYCLING is very good for your heart.

D = DANCING is a fantastic way of moving around.

E = ENERGY builds through exercise – energy makes energy.

F = FUN movement is the best movement.

G = GARDENING is a good mild exercise and so healthy.

H = HYDRO POWER to stronger bones through exercise.

I = INTENSITY in exercise is good to lower your blood pressure.

J = JOGGING on a treadmill or in a field to get the heart rate up.

K = KICKBOXING gets you fit and helps with self-defence skills.

L = LIFTING weights, or gentle lifting of your own body weight.

M = MEDITATION relax deep and breath into your movements.

N = "NO!" is what you say to your excuses.

O = OUTDOOR LIFE: It is so good for your heath to be outside.

P = PILATES very good for your core strength and flexibility.

Q = QUIT? Never!

R = RUNNING: Have good footwear and a sports bra.

S = SWIMMING No better exercise for people with MS.

T = TENNIS is fun and great for keeping fit!

U= UNIQUE is your self-expression of movement.

V = VITAMINS to boost your bodies strength, so take them.

W = WALKING is the most useful exercise in this world.

X= XTREAM SPORTS are not needed. Don't get hurt. just move!

Y = YOGA will both relax and strengthen you.

Z = ZUMBA: a jamming dance fitness class.

The point of the above list is to get you thinking. There is more than one way to get to a mountain top. It is up to you to determine which path is best suited for your body type, personality, and current capacity.

The chief goal is to have fun. If it is not fun to you, you probably will not do it but if it *is* fun for you, then no one can stop you. Your path to increased activity can be simple. Walk rather than drive. Take stairs if you can. Hike or do marital arts or work in the garden.

It does not matter, just keep moving. A key indicator of death is lack of movement. If you are alive (and would prefer to stay that way) we've got to get it moving so start this day. You will feel so much better when you do. Starting to move and exercise is a key component of breaking the chains of MS.

Get yourself free.

MS does not own you!

***

14: ADDITIONAL RESOURCES

Multiple Sclerosis Organizations:

UK

MS SOCIETY – MS NATIONAL CENTRE.
372 Edgeware Road
London
NW2 6ND
Website: https://www.mssociety.org.uk
Helpline # 0800-800-8000

Clinics & Doctors:

UK

OXYGEN THERAPY CENTRE
Unit 8, Park Road Industrial Estate,
Swanley, Kent. BR8 8AH
Tel: 01322-663042.
Website: http://www.swanleytherapycentre.org

USA

NATIONAL MULTIPLE SCLEROSIS SOCIETY
Various Locations in the USA
Website: https://www.nationalmssociety.org
Hotline # 1-800-344-4867

HANGER CLINIC
Various Locations in the USA
Website: http://www.hangerclinic.com
Information Toll Free # 1-877-442-6437
DOCTOR PRAKASH DESAI
MS CONSULTANT
3565 Del Amo Blvd, Suite 200.
Torrance.
CA90503
USA
Telephone # 1-310-214-0811

RECOMMENDED BOOKS:

MS Related

A Health Professional's Guild Dietary Supplements and Multiple Sclerosis
by Allan C. Bowling M.D. PhD

Mild Movement Exercises Helpful for MS

Qigong: The Quick & Easy Start Up Guide
by Frank Blaney

Inspiration

The Mystery of Belief: How to Manifest Your Dreams
by Christopher Dines

More Information from Maria Ann Laver:

https://www.instagram.com/maria_ann_laver
https://www.facebook.com/AuthorMariaAnnLaver

***

ABOUT THE AUTHOR

For 30 years Maria Ann Laver was a successful Number One sales woman in the United Kingdom. She maintained her amazingly successful career even while being pregnant four times (with some miscarriages), enduring a separation, raising two children, and overcoming many tremendous challenges.

In the midst of Maria's productive life she was suddenly stricken with Multiple Sclerosis. From the ravages of this dreadful disease she endured blindness, intense fatigue, disability and compromised mobility. She decided to *fight back*, determined to prevail against the mysterious and disabling disease of MS.

Maria is quick to affirm she is not a doctor or medical professional. She does not dictate medical advice to MS sufferers. She is simply sharing her amazing personal path to victory over the symptoms of MS. She is passionate about empowering others to take control of their health and lifestyle.

Maria's conviction is that our bodies are a reflection of our lifestyle choices. Determined 'not to be owned' by MS and to live a life free of blindness, disability, and dependence upon medication, she integrated *natural lifestyle choices* into her daily routines. She has pulled back her life from the grips of MS. As an author and speaker she is vibrantly passionate about inspiring others with her personal transformation and pragmatic tips to achieve health and well-being.

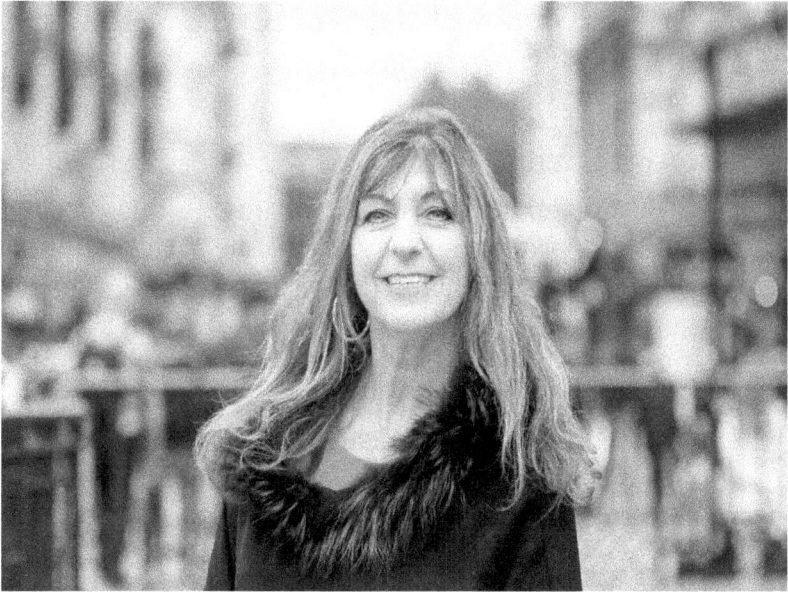

HANDCRAFTED HEALTHY, DELICIOUS AND EASY REJUVENATION RECIPES

By Maria Ann Laver

Food Is Our Best Friend for Health & Healing. In this complementary section, I share just a brief sample of some of the recipes I have handcrafted and created myself. These recipes were designed by me to match the healthy lifestyle eating tips that I write about in this book, *MS You Don't Own Me*. Each one I have created myself and I prepare and eat daily. They are tried and true. In this book I share my background as a professional chef and I love to cook. It is one of my all-time favourite activities. So, as I was forced to go through my personal health challenges I decided to fight the symptoms of Multiple Sclerosis (MS) naturally – using food. Food can be our medicine or our poison. The choice is up to us.

We all love to eat and just as we can get sick from what we eat, we can also get healthier from what we choose to eat. Many people have the very mistaken idea that healthy food equals bad tasting food. Ridiculous! These recipes are not only healthy, they all taste great, and all of them are very easy to prepare. Struggling with an illness means we do not have a lot of energy or time so these recipes are handcrafted with that reality in mind. We are planning on coming out with a full-on cookbook soon, as a sequel to 'MS You Don't Own Me' so, let us know what kind of recipes you would like more of. We would love get your input! Please enjoy these delicious recipes as a complimentary gift of thanks from me. I share my cooking with family and friends as a gift of love. I share these recipes with you in the same spirit. I wish I could come into each of your homes and cook for you! But instead, I have created this recipe booklet for you to try some out. I love eating them, as does my family... I think you will also. They are easy to prepare, so go for it! To begin, just try one recipe, once a week. If you are interested in getting more, please just contact me on Instagram or Facebook. Let me know what you think!

https://www.instagram.com/maria_ann_laver
https://www.facebook.com/AuthorMariaAnnLaver

BREAKFAST

AVOCADO ON TOAST – QUICK BREAKFAST

Great for your brain to start your day. Great for your heart to turn up the heat to start the digestive metabolism. It is quick, tasty, and provides healthy fats for your day.

INGREDIENTS

1 x small avocado skinned with stone removed

1 x tiny bit of chopped red and green fresh chilli

touch of black pepper

touch of pink sea salt

1 to 2 slices of organic 'Ezekiel' sprouted bread

DIRECTIONS

Take the cut and peeled avocado and put in a bowl. Smash slightly with a fork.

Pop one or two slices of 'Ezekiel' brand organic sprouted bread (available in most stores) into the toaster and toast. Mix together the avocado with black cracked pepper and salt. Spread it on top of toasted organic Ezekiel bread. Sprinkle on top of the toast and avocado mixture a touch of fresh chopped red and green chillies. Easy to prepare, great tasting, and such a healthy breakfast. Just eat and enjoy!

***

ORGANIC JUMBO OATS WITH 'ASHWAGANDHA'

I use always a tiny amount of traditional organic herbs each day for added strength and health. Ashwagandha is a traditional medicinal herb from India and is used extensively in Ayurveda. It is an herb which is an 'adaptive', which means its healing properties adjust somewhat to your specific body type and conditions.

Ashwagandha has many health benefits. It is energizing, calming, a restorative, good for your brain and overall strength. With all these added benefits it can improve your quality of life and help boost brain function. We can all use a little more of that! Ashwagandha is easy to use in a powder form. You can get it in some Indian grocery stores, or look for the herb online. It also comes in pills, but you want the plain raw powder. It cost less that way and you can use it as an addition to smoothies or in this delicious breakfast dish.

INGREDIENTS

1 x large dab of natural fat free yogurt or dairy free yogurt

40g organic jumbo oats

¼ teaspoon organic Ashwagandha powder

1 teaspoon chia seeds

¼ teaspoon wheatgrass powder (an iron rich superfood)

¼ teaspoon Spirulina powder (superfood powder, great source of protein)

DIRECTIONS

In covered saucepan cook the 40 g of organic jumbo oats according the package directions. Allow to cool a bit when cooked before you add the other ingredients. Mix all above ingredients together in the saucepan. Then add this mixture to small plastic containers with lids. Place the containers in the refrigerator overnight with the lids on. In the morning, empty the container into a serving bowl (or take the container to work if you are on the go). Top with frozen mixed berries like cherries or blueberries. You can also dribble a small amount of natural honey on top for a little extra sweetness and energy.

***

LUNCH OR DINNER MEALS

SWEET POTATO CURRY

Saturated fat free. Serve with steamed vegetables, Serves 4. Cooking time 45 minutes.

Preheat Oven Gas 7, Electric 220c or Fan 200c

INGREDIENTS

450g x sweet potato peeled and diced into small cubes (approx. ½ inch cubes)

3 x red bell peppers, with seeds removed (dice up two peppers then finely slice the third)

3 x garlic cloves finely chopped or minced

1 x medium sized onion

35g of fresh ginger, peeled and chopped

1 x level teaspoon hot paprika

1 x tablespoon fresh chopped red and green chilli

½ teaspoon sprinkle of ground chilli powder (hot!)

1 x teaspoon of ground Tandoori Masala spice mix (made of turmeric, cumin and coriander)

3 x teaspoons mild curry powder

3 x teaspoons of tomato puree

250g baby spinach leaves

1 x handful of chopped fresh coriander

150g fat free natural yogurt, or dairy free yogurt

salt (to taste)

ground black pepper (to taste)

DIRECTIONS

Lightly spray the roasting tray with olive oil cooking spray, then place the diced sweet potatoes and diced peppers together on the tray. Add salt and pepper.

Put into the hot oven for 30 minutes, tossing around at the edges.

Place and heat the frying pan on the top of the cooker, spray with pan spray and add onions and finely chopped pepper for about 10 minutes stirring frequently.

Add the ginger, garlic and all mixed spices.

Stir for 5 minutes until fragrant.

Add 500ml of boiling water from kettle and the tomato puree.

Bring to the boil for 2 minutes, then add the spinach.

Cover the pan, leave to simmer for about 15 minutes, then remove from the heat.

Add the oven roasted potatoes and peppers, yogurt and fresh coriander and stir.

Then it is ready to eat!

***

SCOTTISH HOT SMOKED SALMON & LARGE PRAWN SEAFOOD SALAD

This is a great and tasty lunch or dinner. If you have a guest, break this out and they will rave about how good it is! It is extremely high in healthy proteins and fats. It is filling, satisfying, and you will feel like you are being treated at a fine restaurant to a special meal. But, it is easy to prepare.

Serves 4 people. Ready in 15 minutes!

INGREDIENTS

organic hot smoked salmon slices (smoked over oak wood for a mild smoke)

or, 400g organic poached salmon fillet

large cooked tiger or king prawns

4 x organic free-range eggs

half an iceberg lettuce

small bag rocket leaves

300g sweet cherry tomatoes

large cucumber

organic apple cider vinegar

sea salt and black pepper to taste

DIRECTIONS

Place eggs into boiling water for 5 minutes or so. Drain, run them under cold water and remove the shells. Take the shelled eggs and slice in half and cut the cherry tomatoes in half. Cover the serving plates with iceberg lettuce and rocket leaves (washed). Slice the cucumber and lay over the lettuce

Separate the salmon pieces over the top of the salad

Place 4-5 cooked prawns on top

Add a sprinkle of organic apple cider vinegar over the egg halves

Add a drizzle of dressing (see below), cracked black pepper and sea salt to taste

Dressing:

Small container of Greek natural fat-free yogurt or dairy free yogurt

4 tablespoons fresh dill

4 teaspoons dried mint

1 whole unwaxed lemon, zested and juiced.

Mix the above ingredients in a bowl and trickle over the salad to taste.

Store any remaining dressing in a container in fridge for use as required.

***

GOAT CHEESE POWER SALAD

Healthy, super easy to prepare, and super delicious

INGREDIENTS

goat's cheese of your choice cut into bite size pieces

1x apple coarsely grated

handful of rocket & baby spinach leaves (½ small bag)

50g whole shelled walnuts pieces

50g sultanas

A few chopped fresh chives

200g tin kidney beans or black beans

100g sugar-snap peas

1 x teaspoon Dijon mustard

black pepper to taste

DIRECTIONS

Wash the greens and let drain in a colander. If using canned beans, drain and rinse the beans. Dice up some chives. Mix all the ingredients together in a bowl and plate to suit your fancy. Add the goat's cheese on top and add the dressing to taste. Voilà!

***

HEALTHY SNACKS

SWEET POTATO WEDGES

Sweet potatoes are OK for diabetics. They are better for you than regular potatoes (especially if you suffer from diabetes). They do not convert to sugar in the body as much or as quickly as a normal potato would. They have more vitamins, are slightly sweet, and taste great!

INGREDIENTS

4 x sweet potatoes, or if preferred, use King Edwards or Maris Pipers.

low calorie cooking spray

salt, pepper and vinegar to taste

DIRECTIONS

Take sheets of baking paper and line a baking tray with them. Preheat your oven 200c, Fan 180c / Gas 6.

Take your sweet potatoes and chop them into wedges. Leave them with the skin on (wash well before chopping). Just like normal potatoes you can cook them in boiling salted water for about 6 to 10 minutes. Drain the hot water off through a colander. Leave the boiled sweet potatoes to cool for 5 minutes. Take the flat baking tray lined with the baking paper. Spray with low calorie cooking spray oil. Arrange the chips or wedges flat onto the sprayed baking paper.

Slightly salt and pepper them (not too much, you want to be able to taste the actual sweet potato). You can spray a little of the low-calorie spray light pan spray onto them once they are arranged flat and seasoned.

Bake for 30 minutes until golden brown. Remove from the oven and let them cool. Sprinkle with vinegar if liked. Then simply enjoy these healthy, fat free, but delicious Sweet Potato Wedges.

Still craving more potatoes? They are a big part of the English diet. Here is another healthy option, using regular potatoes.

***

MARMITE ROAST POTATOES

These are a healthier (and quite delicious) version of an old classic.

INGREDIENTS

1lb of King Edward or Maris Piper potatoes
sea salt and black pepper
Marmite spread

DIRECTIONS

Pre heat the oven: 200c electric, 180c fan or gas mark 7.

Peel the potato then cut into quarters

Place into a pan of boiling water and boil for 10 minutes.

Drain and the shake up the cooked potatoes in the pan to 'rough up' the outsides.

Let them sit for 5 minutes with lid on the saucepan.

Add a tablespoon of Marmite over the cut boiled potatoes. Then take the pieces and space out onto a baking tray, sprinkle with salt and ground black pepper.

Roast until the skin is crispy.

***

DRINKS

COCONUT MILK AND TURMERIC WARM 'SLEEPY-TIME' DRINK

With this warm, delicious, sweet drink, you can perhaps get an extra hour of sleep each night – which can help you live longer. This warming drink is also very anti-inflammatory.

INGREDIENTS

2 x cups of coconut milk

I x teaspoon of turmeric (raw root – grated)

approx. 1 x teaspoon fresh ginger grated or a little more if liked

½ teaspoonful of cinnamon

touch of black pepper

pinch of fresh grated nutmeg

natural honey to taste

DIRECTIONS

In a saucepan add the grated turmeric root, fresh ginger, fresh nutmeg, and cinnamon spices. Carefully bring to the boil and then simmer for about 40 minutes. Let it cool, pass through a sieve and enjoy the drink. You can also eat the grated pieces of turmeric and ginger or tip them back into the drink if you wish.

Make sure to use fresh turmeric which comes from the root of the Curcuma longa plant. Turmeric medicine has been used for years in China, and India as a powerful anti-inflammatory. This will help you sleep deeper and bring some alleviation of sore joints.

***

WHAT'S NEXT?

Did you enjoy the recipes? Did you enjoy eating the scrumptious food? Are you interested in getting a cookbook? Let us know as we develop the next sequel to this first book. We are still developing it so your input would be very much appreciated.
Here is to your dynamic health and to a joyous long life ahead!

Love & Blessings,

Maria Ann Laver

***